Diverse Perspectives on Aging in a Changing World

Focusing on under-researched aspects of social, economic and political change, this volume offers fresh insights into aging, older people and their families. It combines an international and interdisciplinary approach. Chapters explore the contexts in which family roles, institutional practices, public policies, and social and cultural discourses evolve, connecting analyses of aging issues and policy development with sound research practices, as well as previously ignored gaps in professional practice.

Topics covered include politics and policy, health and social care, culture and migration, urban and rural sociology, gender studies, technology and economics. The book will be of particular interest to students and researchers in gerontology, community development, geography and population studies, along with researchers and professionals in physiotherapy, nursing and social work.

Gillian Joseph is Director of Clear Pane Research Services in Guelph, Canada, providing leadership to a team of research specialists who undertake independent research and provide research support to professionals, graduate students, academics and community-based researchers. Previously she was Research Associate at the Centre for Families, Work and Well-being at the University of Guelph, and also served as Lecturer at the University of Guelph and the University of Guelph-Humber in Toronto.

Routledge Studies in Health and Social Welfare

Diverse Perspectives on Aging in a Changing World

Edited by Gillian Joseph

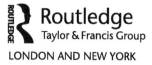
Routledge
Taylor & Francis Group

LONDON AND NEW YORK

First published 2017
by Routledge

2 Park Square, Milton Park, Abingdon, Oxfordshire OX14 4RN
52 Vanderbilt Avenue, New York, NY 10017

Routledge is an imprint of the Taylor & Francis Group, an informa business

First issued in paperback 2020

British Library Cataloguing-in-Publication Data
A catalogue record for this book is available from the British Library

Library of *Congress Cataloging-in-Publication Data*
Names: Joseph, Gillian, editor.
Title: Diverse perspectives on aging in a changing world / edited by Gillian Joseph.
Description: London : Routledge, 2017. | Series: Routledge studies in health and social welfare ; 14 | Includes bibliographical references and index.
Identifiers: LCCN 2016019698| ISBN 9781138195479 (hbk) | ISBN 9781315638386 (ebk)
Subjects: LCSH: Aging--Social aspects. | Aging--Economic aspects. | Older people--Social conditions. | Population aging.
Classification: LCC HQ1061 .D575 2017 | DDC 305.26--dc23
LC record available at https://lccn.loc.gov/2016019698

ISBN: 978-1-138-19547-9 (hbk)
ISBN: 978-0-367-59595-1 (pbk)

Typeset in Sabon
by GreenGate Publishing Services, Tonbridge, Kent

To my mother, a geriatric nurse, who showed me the incredible beauty that still lingers in a tree that has finished blooming

Contents

Illustrations

Figures

Tables

Contributors

Carol Anderson has a clinical background in emergency and cardiovascular/critical care nursing as well as extensive administrative experience in tertiary, rural and territorial health centres, including Director of Patient Care Informatics at the Royal Alexandra Hospital in Edmonton, Canada. As the Principal of CA Consulting, she obtained private-sector experience in the field of Telehealth (provincially, nationally and internationally) as well as in Seniors Care management. She combined these experiences to help inform municipal, provincial and federal governments in Canada about needs in informatics and seniors' healthcare. She was also a sessional instructor with Athabasca University in Canada.

Katherine W. Bauer is an Assistant Professor in the Department of Nutritional Sciences at the University of Michigan School of Public Health. She received her PhD in Epidemiology with a specialization in Behavioral Epidemiology from the University of Minnesota and a MS in Health and Social Behavior from the Harvard School of Public Health. Her research focuses on identifying social and behavioral determinants of obesity during childhood and adolescence, and the translation of such etiologic research into feasible and effective community-based interventions. Much of her work focuses on the role of families in children's and adolescents' nutrition behaviors and obesity risk including understanding 1) how the family environment influences children's obesogenic behavior; 2) how contextual factors and socio-economic stressors affect weight-related parenting and the family environment; and 3) how to engage vulnerable families in obesity prevention efforts.

Sandy Bell is the Manager of Patient Care at Deer Lodge Centre, on the Chronic Care Respiratory unit. Responsibilities include facilitating and supporting excellence in care through the collaboration of an interdisciplinary leadership team in a long term care setting. Prior to this, she spent three and a half years at St. Boniface General Hospital as Director of Family Medicine, Rehab/Geriatrics and Palliative Care leading core programs such as Falls Prevention and Care of Older Persons facility wide. For 13 years she was the Director of Quality, Patient Safety, Clinical Risk Management and Education Services at Misericordia Health Centre in Winnipeg, as well as a Nursing Instructor for over 17 years. During the course of her career, she has spent countless hours advocating for vision care for older persons who reside in the long term care setting. Her research, publications and presentations, highlight a lack of access to vision care services for this population group. She was instrumental in developing and lobbying for permanent funding for a vision care program for seniors who reside in the long term care setting in Manitoba. Her research indicates that improving vision in this population group, decreases falls and injuries as well as improves quality of life. She continues to advocate programming for seniors at Deer Lodge Centre and currently is participating in the initiation of the creation of standards for Continuing Complex Care which includes falls and injury prevention and health promotion strategies.

*Lori D. Campbell is Associate Professor in the Departments of Sociology and Health, Aging and Society, and Associate Dean (Academic) in the Faculty of Social Sciences, McMaster University, Hamilton, Canada. Her research expertise is primarily in the area of aging and family: masculinity and men's roles and experiences in filial caregiving; inheritance and family relationships; and adult sibling ties in middle and later life. She is the principal investigator on a SSHRC-funded qualitative study that explores the experience and meaning of inheritance within families, and is co-lead investigator on research that examines the use of therapy dogs on campus for university students' well-being. She is the co-author of a Canadian textbook on aging, with publications in family and aging journals.

Michael P. Carroll is Professor in the Department of Sociology at Wilfrid Laurier University, Waterloo, Canada and he has served as Dean of Arts at Laurier. He is well known internationally for his historical studies of popular Catholicism in Italy, Ireland and New Mexico. In addition to his work on religion, however, Carroll has co-published (with Lori Campbell) a number of articles on the ways in which sons providing care to older parents perform gender. Prior to coming to Laurier, he was a Sociology Professor at Western (then the University of Western Ontario), where he served as Chair of Sociology and President of Western's Faculty Association. Carroll has authored seven books, more than 65 peer-reviewed articles, and numerous reviews and solicited articles.

Maiga Chang is Associate Professor in the School of Computing Information and Systems, Athabasca University, Canada. His research mainly focuses on mobile learning and ubiquitous learning, museum e-learning, game-based learning, educational robots, learning behavior analysis, data mining, intelligent agent technology, computational intelligence in e-learning and mobile healthcare.

Kristin Crawford completed her Bachelor of Science in Psychology degree at Trent University in Peterborough, Canada, followed by the Research Analyst Program at Georgian College. She joined Charlton Strategic Research in Toronto, Canada, in 2007. Now a senior research analyst, she manages projects in a variety of categories, including video consumption, telecommunications, event experience and satisfaction and fan segmentation, as well as syndicated sport sponsorship studies around the Olympics, NHL, MLB and NBA.

Nora Cristall is a licensed social worker with over 30 years of experience in social work in healthcare. Her experience includes several years in healthcare leadership and evaluation. Her research involves examining differences in health outcomes considering neighborhood area indicators of deprivation. This involves multilevel, multivariate analyses of neighborhood indicators in combination with clinical data. Having training in both qualitative and quantitative research, she has participated in a range of projects involving access to services. This includes homelessness and alternative settings for recovery of more marginalized groups, the transition of youth with disabilities to the adult family services system and complex care planning for older residents of the north-east sector of Winnipeg, Canada. Current research interests focus on aging and poverty issues, such as health equity and pension reform. She is a past board member of the Manitoba Association of Registered Social Workers and was an active editor for the Associations Newsletter *Prairie Ink* for many years. She has taught as a lecturer with the University of Manitoba Faculty of Social Work. Her teaching includes topics on research and evaluation as well as Canadian social welfare policy.

***Adam Davey** is a Developmental Psychologist with training in Human Development and Family Studies from the Pennsylvania State University. He is Associate Dean for Research in the College of Health Sciences at the University of Delaware. Previously, he was Professor and Founding Chair of the Department of Epidemiology and Biostatistics in Temple University's College of Public Health, Senior Research Scientist at the Polisher Research Institute and Associate Professor at the University of Georgia. His research addresses issues of marital and intergenerational relationships, family caregiving and comparative analysis of the interface between formal and informal care networks, particularly in the United States, Great Britain and Sweden. Currently, he is examining regional variability in how families have responded to changes over a six-year period in the availability of formal services across Sweden. He also collaborates on projects investigating longitudinal changes in care networks within families and couples' navigation of the retirement process.

***Lee Anne Davies** has extensive experience in the financial industry which resulted in her interest in financial issues for aging populations as a public health issue. She completed her doctoral studies on the topic of poverty and financial capability in adults age 55+ with supervisor John Hirdes at the University of Waterloo, Canada. The analysis of financial abilities and economic trade-offs of this population was the first of its kind using inter-RAI data. Three provincial jurisdictions were studied. The relationships of poverty and financial capability with demographic, health, social and life-style factors resulted in new insights and recommendations for government and private sector policy considerations. These results also inspired her to found and continue her work through Agenomics.ca in Victoria, Canada, and to pursue issues of autonomy and privacy in an ageing population.

Margaret Edwards is Dean of the Faculty of Health Disciplines, Athabasca University, Canada. Her areas of research interest include innovative online teaching strategies and exemplary online teaching practices. She also explores issues related to older adult caregivers and their care recipients. She is a registered nurse and holds a PhD in Educational Policy and Administrative Studies at the University of Calgary, Canada.

****Brian K. Gran** is Associate Professor in the Department of Sociology, Law School, and Mandel School of Applied Social Sciences of Case Western Reserve University, Cleveland, Ohio, USA. A former lawyer, Gran's research focuses on human rights and institutions that support and hinder their enforcement, with a particular interest in whether law can intervene into private spheres. With David Brunsma and Keri Iyall Smith, he edited *The Handbook of Sociology and Human Rights*. A co-founder of the ASA Human Rights section, he serves on the Steering Committee and Council of the Science and Human Rights Project of the American Association for the Advancement of Science. He is former President of the thematic group on Global Justice and Human Rights of the International Sociological Association. For his research on independent children's rights institutions, Gran enjoyed support from the US National Science Foundation, as well as a Visiting Fellowship of the Swiss National Science Foundation and as a Fulbright Scholar to Iceland. Gran is a member of the U.S. National Conference of Lawyers and Scientists. He is affiliated with the Case Western University Center on Aging and Health.

****Pamela Hawranik** has been with the University of Athabasca in Canada since June 2008 when she was appointed the first Dean of Graduate Studies. Prior to this, she was Associate Dean in the Faculty of Graduate Studies, and Associate Dean for graduate programs at the Faculty of Nursing at the University of Manitoba, Winnipeg, Canada. She is also currently Research Affiliate at the Centre on Aging and Adjunct Professor at the Faculty of Nursing, both at the University of Manitoba. She held an academic position at the Faculty of Nursing for 18 years and taught both the undergraduate and graduate programs, as well as courses that were on-site and courses that were offered by blended delivery. Prior to joining the University of Manitoba, she held a number of positions: Clinical Nurse Specialist, Geriatric Medicine, St. Boniface Hospital;

Executive Director for a non-profit community nursing agency; policy analyst for Manitoba Health; and a Public Health Nurse and Home Care Case coordinator in rural Manitoba. She has recently co-authored a book that is currently in press entitled: *Context and its Influence on the Spread and Uptake of Evidence within Alberta North Zone Home Care Centres.* She has published a significant number of peer-reviewed papers as well as academic reports and book chapters. Her clinical background informs her research in gerontology as she examines the effectiveness of community services in meeting the needs of older adults and their unpaid caregivers. She has been an investigator for several nationally funded studies identifying the barriers and issues in delivering and accessing home care services in rural Canada. Several studies have also evaluated various interventions on the health of older adults, such as alternative therapies and vision care services.

Gord Hendren is President and CEO of Charlton Strategic Research, a Toronto-based boutique insights and marketing solutions company with an international perspective in Canada. The company provides strategically relevant insights and strategic marketing direction to add value to clients' businesses. The client base spans many industry categories including: media, broadcast, online, events, social media, satellite radio, telecommunications, technology, financial services, automotive, petroleum, airline, retail, athletic equipment and others. Given this experience, he is a recognized expert in brand marketing and brand health. In the course of his business, he conducts research analytics on all age groups from pre-school to seniors. He is a member of ESOMAR (an international association of research insights professionals) and a guest lecturer at Queen's University School of Business, Kingston, Canada.

John P. Hirdes is Professor in the School of Public Health and Health Systems, University of Waterloo, Canada. He is also Professor in the School of Public Health and Health Systems at the University of Waterloo. He is the senior Canadian Fellow and a Board Member of interRAI, an international consortium of researchers from over 35 countries. He chairs interRAI's International Network for Mental Health and the interRAI Network of Canada. He is also Fellow of the Canadian Academy of Health Sciences. He has over 190 publications in peer-reviewed journals and academic book chapters. His primary areas of interest include geriatric assessment, mental health, healthcare and service delivery, case mix systems, quality measurement, health information management and quantitative research methods. In 2012, he received the University of Waterloo Award for Excellence in Graduate Supervision. In addition, he received the Queen Elizabeth II Diamond Jubilee Medal through the Canadian Home Care Association and the Canadian Association on Gerontology.

*Gillian Joseph is Editor of this book and Director of Clear Pane Research Services in Guelph, Canada. She has a Master of Science degree in Family Relations and Human Development with a specialization in Gerontology from the University of Guelph, Canada. She began her academic career at Guelph in the mid-1990s through the Canadian Aging Research Network (CARNET). Prior to her work as Director of Clear Pane Research Services, she was Research Associate at the Centre for Families, Work & Well-being at the University of Guelph for eight years, undertaking research independently and in partnership with leading academics and practitioners across Canada. She explored topics associated with family caregiving, institutional long-term care, home care work, aboriginal eldercare, work/family balance, mental health and elder abuse. She has also served as a lecturer at the University of Guelph and the University of Guelph Humber, Toronto, teaching courses in social gerontology, family relations, program evaluation and social policy. She has over 25 publications in peer-reviewed and professional journals and has authored or co-authored several book chapters and a number of research reports for leading research funding agencies. In 1996, she edited an international monograph on issues associated with aging that was published by the University of Guelph. She has served as a member of the Mission and Ethics Subcommittee of the Board of St. Joseph's Health Centre in Guelph, as a member of the Waterloo/Wellington Coordinated Gerontology Education Strategy and the Waterloo/Wellington Dementia Network. She also served as Research Chair on the Board of the Ontario Caregiving Coalition for several years. She has been Director of Clear Pane Research Services for the past seven years, providing leadership to a team of research specialists who develop and teach research methodology programs to graduate students and professionals, as well as providing support and services to academic and community-based researchers. Currently, she is working on a number of independent research projects with academics across Canada on a variety of topics, including seniors and the environment, the impact of weather on front-line institutional caregiving, respite experiences of employed family caregivers and caregiving policy.

Dr Kinshuk holds the NSERC/CNRL/Xerox/McGraw Hill Chair for Adaptivity and Personalization in Informatics. He is also Full Professor in the School of Computing and Information Systems and Associate Dean of Faculty of Science and Technology at Athabasca University, Canada. Areas of research interests include learning analytics, learning technologies; mobile, ubiquitous and location aware learning systems; and cognitive profiling and interactive technologies.

Linda Chiu Wa Lam is a Physician, Professor and Chair of the Department of Psychiatry, Director of the Dementia Research Unit and Director of the Chen Wai Vivien Foundation of Therapeutic Physical and Mental Exercise Centre at the Chinese University of Hong Kong. Her research interests include early detection and intervention of mild cognitive impairment and dementia, and biomarker evaluations for mild cognitive impairment and dementia. She also engages in research on determinants of healthy aging and the epidemiology of mental disorders in Hong Kong. She is past President of the Hong Kong College of Psychiatrists and Founding President of the Chinese Dementia Research Association, as well as past Chief Editor of the *East Asia Archives of Psychiatrists*.

Belinda Leach is Associate Dean (Research) and former Acting Dean for the College of Social & Applied Human Sciences at the University of Guelph, as well as Professor of Anthropology. Her major research interests concern changes in livelihoods in restructuring economies at the turn of the twenty-first century. She has examined the implications of shifts in the organization of work and how families and individuals accommodate and resist changing work patterns, through decisions around migration, care and employment. She led an SSHRC-funded Community-University Research Alliance (CURA), Rural Women Making Change (2005–2010), as well as several other SSHRC-funded projects. She has published extensively in peer-reviewed journals and contributed chapters to books on topics associated with women, work and health. She is co-author of *Contingent Labour, Disrupted Lives: Labour and Community in the New Rural Economy* (University of Toronto Press, 2002) with Tony Winson, which received the 2003 John Porter Memorial Book Prize from the Canadian Sociology and Anthropology Association. She has co-edited four books, and has served as Anthropology Editor of the *Canadian Review of Sociology and Anthropology* and co-editor of *Identities: Global Studies in Culture and Power*. She is a founding member of the University of Guelph's Centre for Families, Work and Well-being and Institute for Community Engaged Scholarship.

Shelly Kin Shan Leung has a Master of Science degree in Cognitive Neuroscience from University College London. Upon graduation in 2011, she joined the research team in the Department of Psychiatry at The Chinese University of Hong Kong. She was the main researcher executing large-scale research on mild cognitive impairment and dementia in elderly populations and she also engaged in the Hong Kong Mental Morbidity Survey epidemiology study. She completed a Postgraduate Certificate in Psychology at the University of Hong Kong in 2013. Since then, she has been working as a Research Associate in the Department of Psychology at the University of Hong Kong, teaching Biological Psychology, Perception, Cognitive Science and Statistics. Her current research interests include clinical and neurological factors in aging and dementia.

Roger Mannell is a psychologist and Distinguished Professor Emeritus of Leisure Studies and Past Dean of the Faculty of Applied Health Sciences, University of Waterloo, Canada. He was also Director of the RBC

Retirement Research Centre. He is a recipient of the US National Parks and Recreation Association's Theodore and Franklin Roosevelt Research Excellence Award. His research interests include the social psychology of leisure, aging, lifestyle and health, work and leisure, program evaluation and research methods.

Donnie McIntosh is Principal at McIntosh Health Care Consulting and a Clinical Gerontology Consultant with Athabasca University, Canada. For the past 20 years, her nursing career has spanned the areas of acute care, community health, research, education, human milk banking and eldercare.

Beth Perry is Professor in the Centre for Nursing and Health Studies, Faculty of Health Disciplines, Athabasca University, Canada. Her areas of research include exemplary nursing care of older adults and palliative populations, compassion fatigue in older adult caregivers and career fulfillment of nurses. She is a registered nurse and completed her PhD at the University of Alberta, Edmonton, Canada.

*Valerie Powell has worked as a Psychogeriatric Resource Consultant in Simcoe County, Canada, for over ten years with a home office at Collingwood General and Marine Hospital in Collingwood, Canada. For the past three years, she has been the Behavioral Support System Coordinator in North Simcoe Muskoka, working out of Waypoint Centre for Mental Health Care, Penetanguishene. Prior to this, she was Lecturer at Georgian College, Barrie, Ontario, Instructor at the University of Guelph, Executive Director of the Alzheimer Society of Guelph Wellington and Executive Director of the Georgian Bay Lung Association. She has a Master of Science degree in Family Relations and Human Development with a specialization in Gerontology from the University of Guelph, Canada. She has consulted and provided education to long-term care homes and community agencies and contributed to the work of the Dementia and Elder Abuse Networks. She co-created the "Me & U-First Guide" for people with dementia and the "Me & U-First" online learning program. As a member of the Seniors Health Regional Action Group of the North Simcoe-Muskoka Local Health Integration Network (LHIN), she contributed to the vision for seniors care in North Simcoe Muskoka, and she advocates for improved care on local and provincial seniors, mental health, dementia and behavioral task groups and committees. As well as her roles as practitioner and academic, she has twice been the federal candidate for the Green Party in Simcoe North. Because of her extensive knowledge of and contribution to seniors, she also serves as both Seniors Critic and Mental Health Critic in the Green Party's Shadow Cabinet.

Oi Ling Siu is Professor and Chair of the Department of Applied Psychology at Lingnan University, Hong Kong. Her research interests are in

Occupational Health Psychology, specifically occupational stress, psychology of safety and work–life balance. In the past few years, she has been awarded many of the Research Grants Coucil's General Research Funds (previously Earmarked Research Grants) from the National Natural Science Foundation (China), the Australian Research Council, the Quality Education Fund and research grants from the Occupational Safety & Health Council. She received the Research Excellence Award in May 2002 and the Dr. and Mrs. James Wu Awards for Outstanding Service by Lingnan University in March 2002. She was also awarded the Committee Member of Chinese Association of Employee Assistance Program (EAP) & Organizational Health in November 2004 and received a Guest Professorship at the Graduate School of Chinese Academy of Sciences, PRC, which she has held since 2008. She is Editor of the *International Journal of Stress Management* and the Associate Editor of the *Journal of Occupational Health Psychology.*

*Gina Sylvestre is Assistant Professor of Geography at the University of Winnipeg, Manitoba, Canada. Prior to her position as Assistant Professor, she worked as Research Associate at the Institute of Urban Studies, University of Winnipeg. Her research interests include: transitions in transportation usage by older adults, neighborhood deprivation and aging, and leadership development and knowledge mobilization of rural seniors. She is also connected to the University of Manitoba Centre on Aging. She has published her work in several peer-reviewed journals. Her most recent research has been the exploration of aging in poverty in Winnipeg's North End. Through community immersion and participant observation, she is unfolding the many meanings of growing old in an environment where systematic processes do not afford the informal and formal resources required to age well. She has also collaborated for several years with the Transportation Options Network for Seniors Community Coalition (formerly the Seniors Transportation Working Group) to pursue the issue of mobility and identify those elements in the community that create barriers, as well as best practices that improve transportation for an aging population. With funding from the provincial Healthy Aging and Seniors Secretariat and the Public Health Agency of Canada, she has developed a research program to inform both policy and transport provision for older adults in Manitoba. The program is directed to facilitate community dialogue around improved ways of collaborating and providing mobility services to persons experiencing difficulty in participating fully in both rural and urban communities.

Maximilliane E. Szinovacz has research interests that include families in later life, family caregiving, retirement, grand-parenthood, intergenerational relationships and transfers. Prior to joining the University of Massachusetts, Boston, USA, she served as the Sue Faulkner Scribner Distinguished Professor in Geriatrics at the Glennan Center for Geriatrics and Gerontology, Eastern Virginia Medical School, Norfolk, USA. She has also held faculty and research positions at Old Dominion University, University of Illinois, Florida State University and Pennsylvania State University. She has consulted on projects with the American Association of Retired Persons (AARP), European Centre for Social Welfare Policy and Research (Vienna, Austria) and Netherlands Interdisciplinary Demographic Institute, among others. She is a fellow at the National Council on Family Relations and the Gerontological Society of America, and has earned numerous research grants from the National Institute on Aging, AARP, Andus Foundation and Hartford Foundation.

Margaret Waltz is a Postdoctoral Research Associate at the Center for Genomics and Society at the University of North Carolina at Chapel Hill. Her research explores issues associated with medical sociology, gender, social inequality and the media. She completed her PhD at Case Western Reserve University.

*****Blossom Wigdor** is Professor Emerita at the University of Toronto, Canada, and author of the Foreword written for this book. She is the founding Director of what is now called the Institute for Life Course and Aging at the University of Toronto—the first centre for aging of its kind in Canada. In recognition of her accomplishments, she received the Order of Canada in 1989 for "working tirelessly to foster research and education in the problems of aging and to improve the circumstances of the elderly" (Holden, 1989). She was also the founder of the Canadian Association of Gerontology and the first editor of the *Canadian Journal of Aging*. She has published an impressive list of books and articles, including *Canadian Gerontological Collection, Handbook on Mental Health and Aging, Planning Your Retirement: The Complete Canadian Self-help Guide*, and co-authored *The Over-Forty Society: Issues for Canada's Aging Population*. She began her career in the field of clinical psychology. Now, at the age of "90-something," she still engages in research and continues to move beyond the boundaries that defined her as a pioneering academic of our times.

*Contributing authors to the 1996 monograph.

Reference

Holden, A. (1989, January 31). Ahead of her time: All about Blossom Wigdor. *Toronto Star*, D1.

Foreword

There have been many changes in perspectives on aging over the past 20 years, as the world has changed both politically and technologically. Globalization and instant communication have impacted on social policy and on our daily lives. The changing demographic structure of western developed countries, where baby boomers are reaching retirement age, has resulted in issues related to aging becoming more dominant, though many of these issues have not changed over the years. There has been increased diversity in the ethnic and cultural populations, and also in the structure of families, the stability of relationships, economic opportunities and increased geographic mobility. The various chapters in this book reflect these diversities, but also the fact that such issues as healthcare, intergenerational relations, home care and gender issues are still primary concerns.

The changes over the past 20 years have been dramatic in many ways. Economic changes for the elderly are reflected in the increase of the average income for seniors. The fact that more women have been in the work force and thus have pensions has had a huge impact. However, other changes in the labour market have led to fewer people having defined benefit pensions and long-term careers. This suggests that many will be more dependent on government involvement. Technology has changed communication modes and the workplace, impacting older workers, retirement plans and seniors' lives.

The graduate students of 20 years ago have gone on to responsible and prestigious positions, many in academia. Most have stayed in the field of aging. Now, as authors of this book, they find themselves in diverse work situations, and offer thoughtful and wide-ranging insights into relevant issues both from an international and Canadian perspective.

Blossom Wigdor (CM., PhD.), Professor Emerita, University of Toronto, Canada, and Founding Director of the Institute for Life Course and Aging, University of Toronto, Canada

Acknowledgments

There are, of course, many people who shape a project like this along the way. However, some must certainly be recognized here for their significant contributions. First and foremost, my sincere thanks to the authors and co-authors of the various chapters in the book, especially to those who contributed to the monograph 20 years ago and who agreed enthusiastically to return to be part of this project. From an important historical perspective, I would also like to acknowledge the financial support and guidance of Dr. Donna Woolcott who, as Chair of the Department of Family Studies at the University of Guelph in 1996, made it possible for us to come together as authors in the first place.

To my dear friend and mentor for over 20 years, Dr. Blossom Wigdor, a pioneer and giant in the field of gerontology in Canada, who has graciously come out of a long and busy retirement to write the foreword for this book: we are privileged to have your contribution.

I would particularly like to acknowledge Emily Briggs, our first Associate Editor at Routledge on this project, whose keen response to our proposal, quick turnaround on e-mails, sound advice and patience was greatly appreciated—and to the new team at Routledge to whom the baton has been passed. Many thanks.

It is also important to acknowledge the funders of some of the research reported in this volume—the range of government, university, funding agencies, foundations and private-sector sponsors that have provided financial support for our work. Their support speaks volumes to the importance of recognizing the reciprocal relationship between research and professional practice, and its value and relevance for older people, their families and policy-makers around the world. Although not an exhaustive list, we would particularly like to acknowledge Athabasca University Academic Research Fund for supporting the research reported here by Perry et al., and the Fort Garry Legion Poppy Fund, Misericordia Health Centre, CIHR Rural Net and Manitoba Health that supported the research reported by Hawranik et al. Thanks also needs to be extended to the Cable and Telecommunications Association for Marketing (CTAM) Canada and the Government of the Hong Kong SAR's Department of Health for providing access to data for the research reported by Hendren et al. and Leung et al., respectively. To the research assistants who assisted us in searching for articles, books and other bits of information, as well as endlessly updating bibliographic software files, we also say "thank you," especially to Merin Valiyaparampil at the University of Guelph.

Last, but most importantly to me, I acknowledge the incredible support that I received from my husband, Alun, over the past year. Tirelessly he assumed the roles of caretaker, housekeeper, chef, idea sounding board and sometimes therapist. In the words of Robert Browning: *Grow old along with me! The best is yet to be…*

Introduction

Gillian Joseph

This book is a collection of original chapters that contribute fresh insights to the growing body of literature on aging, older people and their families. Its approach combines international, interdisciplinary and transdisciplinary perspectives. Key differences between government systems and practices in the USA and Canada are teased out, cross-cultural comparisons are made, and important issues associated with aging in Asia and Europe are brought into focus around topics such as health and transmigration. The book also emphasizes its interdisciplinary and transdisciplinary perspectives by bringing to the attention of readers new theories and research methodologies and innovative practices that have only recently been recognized as integral pieces previously left out of the knowledge "puzzle." The topics presented here draw not only on the disciplines of geriatric medicine and community health, but also those of technology, law, human geography, political science and marketing. These are disciplines that, in some cases, have only recently brought issues of aging and families into their purview. For example, several of the chapters discuss the relationship between aging and technology, highlighting its impact on stereotypes, as well as discussing how intergenerational family connections are strengthened, and well-being is improved, as a result of the interaction between human and machine.

Several of the chapters are groundbreaking in their empirical focus on the under-researched context of social, economic and political change, while others use finely honed tools of research inquiry to uncover gaps in professional practice. Some contributors highlight how political ideology shapes the circumstances of everyday life, uncovering the often-hidden agendas associated with access, gender relations, health practices and economic reform. In each case, they seek to uncover the context in which family roles, institutional practices, public policies and social discourses have evolved, while at the same time connecting these observations and analyses to emerging research platforms. Each of the chapters strives to bridge the gap between theory and practice by linking their relatively disparate literatures to what has happened, and is currently happening, to real people in real situations in North America and elsewhere in the world. By presenting the work of practitioners as well as academics, this book provides an opportunity to create a knowledge transfer loop that informs both the theoretical and the applied; a process that is increasingly being identified as a priority by politicians, academics and practitioners (Bellman, 2011). But there is also something else that is very special about this edited volume.

Twenty years ago, in 1996, an advertisement in a Canadian university newsletter brought 12 graduate student authors together from across Canada, the USA and Great Britain to report to a global audience on their gerontology research. The resulting international interdisciplinary monograph entitled *Difficult Issues in Aging in Difficult Times* (ISBN 088955451X) was published by the University of Guelph in Canada and also became the focus of a dedicated workshop at the Canadian Association on Gerontology conference in Calgary in 1997. This new book brings eight of these same authors together again, many contributing in partnership with their research colleagues from around the world. The original authors are now academics and/or practitioners who are well established in their own fields and disciplines across North America and beyond. They include Lori D. Campbell from McMaster University, Adam Davey from Temple University, Lee Anne Davies from Agenomics, Brian K. Gran from Case Western Reserve University, Pamela Hawranik from Athasbasca University, Valerie Powell from Waypoint Centre for Mental Health Care, Gina Syvestre from the University of Winnipeg and Gillian Joseph from Clear Pane Research Services. This volume provides the reader with an opportunity to reflect on the many changes that have taken place over the past 20 years—changes not only in traditional research paths and professional practices associated with aging, but also those that have shaped the world and the political, social and economic systems in which older adults and their families experience aging. Changes that have prompted us to ask new questions and to seek new paths to understanding. Dr. Blossom Wigdor, who was awarded an Order of Canada for her leadership in aging research as one of the founding academics of the Centre for Studies on Aging at the University of Toronto, the first centre of its kind in Canada, wrote the Foreword for the 1996 monograph, and, 20 years later, it is our privilege and pleasure to again include a Foreword by Dr. Wigdor.

Many academics and practitioners are only beginning to fully acknowledge that aging is not experienced in the same way by everyone. Furthermore, not everyone views aging and older people in the same way (Chasteen and Cary, 2015; Mitnitski and Rockwood, 2015). Each individual has a unique set of inherited genes, is surrounded by a different physical environment and has different life experiences. This can affect not only physical health, but may also shape actions and prejudices. Such diversity makes the study of aging both fascinating and, at the same time, challenging. *Diverse Perspectives on Aging in a Changing World* brings attention to the importance of a broader, international, interdisciplinary and intersectorial understanding of population aging that is reflective of past trends, yet, at the same time, facilitative of new thinking—conceptually, empirically and practically.

The rapidity of change that has occurred in North America, Europe, Asia and other places around the world over the past 20 years is a result, in part, of shifting health, social and economic policies, evolving practices and demographic changes that have created an attractive laboratory for developing and testing new approaches and ideas. New insights have come from a variety of evolving disciplinary paradigms and professional practices (Joseph et al., 2013). These changes mean that researchers and practitioners need to constantly reflect upon remaining gaps in understanding and to encourage others to consider new perspectives and discoveries. It also suggests the importance of re-orienting ourselves and our institutions towards addressing the needs of individuals as well as the needs of the social and economic systems in which we are all immersed (Kolb, 2014; Leach and Joseph, 2011).

As important as reflection is to the strength of good research and practice, it is also important to broaden the scope of inquiry beyond the paradigms in which researchers feel most comfortable. It has been recognized for some time that interdisciplinary research is an effective tool whose strength lies in its incorporation of different methods and theoretical perspectives to assist researchers to more effectively explore and respond to complex, modern societal issues (Butler, 2011). At first glance, the process of aging does not appear to be complicated in its natural progression. However, the social, political, economic and personal contexts that shape how people experience senescence makes aging "one of the most complex, controversial and widely disputed areas of science" (Zhavoronkov and Cantor, 2011, p. 1). The chapters of this book seek to untangle some of this complexity by exploring issues from a diversity of theoretical and professional perspectives. Where paradigm-based windows of enquiry have thus far been narrow in their vision of aging, these new lenses provide further insights that assist in the building of new knowledge. Where policies and practices sit comfortably in their assumptions, these chapters push the reader by asking challenging questions that unravel complacency.

The chapters are organized into three sections. In the first section, entitled *Aging spaces and the individual*, the distinctive challenges faced by older adults in urban and rural areas are presented, as well as related matters of interest at a more micro level. This includes uncovering some of the sources of ageism that are reinforcing stereotypes, identifying gaps in local policies that affect independence and agency, and highlighting new and innovative ways that technology and exercise can facilitate wellness for an older adult wherever he/she lives. For example, Sylvestre invites the reader to consider how older adults move within and through physical space and highlights how issues of access can shape an individual's experiences associated with aging-in-place. Waltz and Gran engage the reader in exploring the modern concept of digital space by looking at how popular television programs portray aging and older people, while Perry et al. lead the reader further into this domain in a discussion of how increasingly tech-savy older adults are navigating cyberspace to learn about health. Leung and her colleagues look at a more cognitively oriented concept of space in a study of older people in Hong Kong and their self-perceptions of health.

The second section, entitled *Aging families: caregiving and gender*, offers diverse insights into critical aspects of family, private and publically funded care. It includes critiques of emerging political ideologies and changing social systems, and examines how these powerful forces are shaping care relationships. This section compels readers to dig deeper, to ask sometimes uncomfortable questions about the changing roles that men and women are assuming as caregivers and what shapes the choices and transitions that aging families must make. In terms of aging families, Davey et al. push the reader to look beyond the traditional lenses that focus on caregiver research to acknowledge that it is not just a spouse who provides eldercare. Instead, it is often the work of a dynamic family care network taking place—the members of which have not been fully explored by research or noticed by policy-makers. Furthermore, Davey et al. suggest that research that traditionally stops at the end of caregiving is incomplete and needs to continue down the life course trajectory to consider what happens to family caregivers immediately and even long after their caregiving duties have finished. Powell's work about communication between aging parents and their adult children dovetails nicely with the concept of care networks as she highlights some of the factors that cause conflict in aging families. Her personal and professional reflections provide important insights into one of the most meaningful of family relationships. The chapter by Hawranik et al. exposes the gap in vision care services that exists in institutional long-term care. This, along with the strong messages associated with gender and eldercare embedded in the chapters authored by Campbell and Carroll and Joseph and Leach, illustrate respectively how political ideology informs policy (or eliminates it) and how ideology can dramatically shape the experience of aging in families who are seeking support for eldercare. While Campbell and Carroll question assumptions associated with gender equity and caregiving within the texts of internet-based advice fora, Joseph and Leach deconstruct the tenets of neoliberalism and the precariousness associated with transmigrant eldercare work for both provider and recipient of care that is the outcome of an increasingly global political trend.

Finally, while on the one hand Section 3, entitled *Aging and economics* highlights the "catch 22" that is sometimes associated with economic risk, poverty and pension reform, it also serves to remind entrepreneurs about the uniqueness of a rapidly growing aging market and the great potential that lies there. It particularly emphasizes the very sensitive balance between economic security and health. Looking at older adults who are at significant risk of abject poverty, the chapters by Davies et al. and Sylvestre and Cristall invite the reader to consider how older adults become marginalized and are rendered invisible when their economic reality is not recognized, and how that invisibility can exclude older adults from access to essentials such as food, activities and services that, in turn, affects their health and well-being. The chapter by Hendren et al. introduces the reader to the world of the aging consumer and what drives the choices that older people make when they pay for and access digital entertainment. This too is a topic that is not often addressed within the gerontological literature. However, the growing global demographic of aging consumers represents an untapped market with behaviors and preferences that need to be acknowledged and accommodated.

In summary, this book reflects the diversity of an ever-changing world, and showcases new ideas about research and practice that are intrinsic to a contemporary understanding of the experiences of older people and their families. The collection is distinctive in its merging not only of the theoretical and the applied, but also of the historical and the cutting edge—all important aspects of what is considered to be the very heart of the cycle of knowledge formation and its translation into policy and practice.

Whether you are a student, an academic, a policy analyst, a professional in social work, medicine or community service, or just someone who craves a deeper understanding of what shapes the experience of human aging, we invite you to turn the page to begin what will be a fascinating journey.

References

Bellman, L. (2011). Knowledge transfer and the integration of research, policy and practice for patient benefit. *Journal of Research Nursing*, *16*(3), 254–270.

Butler, L.S.T. (2011). Barriers and enablers of interdisciplinary research at academic institutions [Doctoral thesis]. University of Southern Mississippi.

Chasteen, A.L. and Cary, L.A. (2015). Age stereotypes and age stigma: Connections to research on subjective aging. *Annual Review of Gerontology and Geriatrics*, *35*(1), 99–119.

Joseph, G., Skinner, M.W. and Yantzi, N.M. (2013). The weather-stains of care: Interpreting the meaning of bad weather for front-line health care workers in rural long-term care. *Social Science & Medicine*, *91*, 194–201.

Kolb, P. (2014). *Understanding Aging and Diversity: Theories and Concepts*. New York: Routledge.

Leach, B. and Joseph, G. (2011). Rural long-term care work, gender, and restructuring. *Canadian Journal on Aging*, June *30*(2), 211–221.

Mitnitski, A. and Rockwood, K. (2015). Aging as a process of deficit accumulation: Its utility and origin. *Interdisciplinary Topics in Gerontology*, *40*, 85–98.

Zhavoronkov, A. and Cantor, C.R. (2011). Methods for structuring scientific knowledge from many areas related to aging research. *PlusOne*, *6*(7). Accessed 24 June 2015 http://journals.plos.org/plosone/article?id=10.1371/journal.pone.0022597.

Section 1

Aging spaces and the individual

1   Aging and sustainability

Creating a discourse on places of inclusive mobility for the promotion of longevity

Gina Sylvestre

Aging-in-place is considered to be crucial to independence and well-being in later life and an important dimension of the concept of successful aging (Schwanen et al., 2012). When one is able to remain in a familiar place of meaning, identity and attachment, the capacity to adapt to the processes of aging are enhanced. While an older person's continuing inclusion within the neighborhood presupposes the ongoing maintenance of mobility, disconnect exists between policies that promote aging-in-place and the barriers faced by older individuals to remain mobile in urban settings. In this chapter, I propose that for seniors to maintain engagement in their neighborhoods, it is imperative that principles of urban sustainability be broadened to create places that support the mobility of older adults, ensuring the community longevity of this growing population.

Today, many older adults reside in lower-density suburbs, and though they would like to remain in these familiar environments, the predominance of auto-based travel as the principal mobility option may not be an ideal alternative for aging-in-place. In fact, American data suggests that half of those over the age of 65 who are non-drivers are forced to remain at home because transport choices are limited (Dunham-Jones, 2005). Modern urban places were designed at a time when aging was not a primary demographic factor and suburban areas contain physical, social and economic infrastructure that constrains access to resources for seniors. Suburbia is organized to perpetuate a spatial form that discourages walkability and usable public spaces. The inaccessibility of these areas creates social exclusion for the older population and ultimately embodies social inequality (Antoninetti and Garrett, 2012). The question is, how can local governments and other sectors address the mobility needs of seniors to promote inclusive places?

Within the realm of environmental gerontology, there is an absence of linkages with wider theoretical perspectives, specifically in relation to changes affecting older persons in the urban context. Similarly, until now dialogue surrounding urban sustainability has not put forth the benefits of focusing on aging-in-place, despite collective pursuits for social and economic equity, as well as ecological restoration. To more effectively position the aging process in an integrated vision of community, it is essential to synthesize urban sustainability principles with the mobility needs of older adults to counter isolation and enhance quality of life. As a response to the lack of theoretical integration, I offer a mobility-inclusive community plan that proposes a broadened view of the linkages among aging-in-place, mobility and the principles of sustainable urban places.

Key to urban sustainability is the premise of the redesign of infrastructure and development patterns providing a basis for the transformation of liveable places. Principles of sustainability must be framed within the meaning of place for seniors requiring a more comprehensive perspective of the mobility spaces of aging. Such mobility spaces include not only the local neighborhood, but also the more distant spaces that enable older adults to be connected to society's function of inclusion and accessibility. This chapter seeks to offer an enhanced concept of mobility space that informs a definition of sustainability, promotes movement and inclusion in the local context, while also creating connectivity to the expansive opportunities made available to all community members.

Aging and transportation research: a limited inquiry

Mobility is generally defined to be the ability to overcome any type of distance, and it incorporates within it perceptions of proximity and accessibility (Banister and Bowling, 2004; Ziegler and Schwanen, 2011). It is crucial to the continuing independence of elderly persons as the ability to be mobile allows access to desired destinations, social networks and community engagement. Gerontological research has widely established the significance of mobility, demonstrating its linkages to the health and well-being of seniors (Spinney et al., 2009). The relevance of mobility to successful aging is therefore recognized, yet investigation in this area is limited to transportation demands and travel patterns, devoid of any consideration of the reasons for unmet mobility needs or the implications of immobility in an older person's life.

In the past ten years, various disciplines have increasingly focused on the everyday mobility of the aging population (Murray, 2015). Despite this attention to the topic, the research lacks innovation, with the majority of inquiry focusing on variability in trip-making, distance and frequency of travel and the types of travel modes (Fobker and Grotz, 2006; Paez et al., 2007). The research mandate has paid particular attention to the frequency of use of the transport continuum that extends from driving to para-transit services for seniors. While evaluation of the adequacy of these mobility options has occurred (Metz, 2000), exploration from a spatial perspective of the reasons why certain modes are used less is generally omitted from the research agenda. The long distances between residences and destinations in current urban settings preclude walking as a mobility choice and instead position it as a form of physical activity. These low-density environments also create inadequate public transit systems that do not meet the mobility needs of the older population, with long walks to bus stops, infrequent service and the concentration of routes primarily focused on employment, education and business destinations. Though taxi service as an alternative option does provide door-to-door service, most seniors are unable to consider it as a regular form of transport because of its high cost. Furthermore, despite the subsidization of urban para-transit services, this option is generally limited to those seniors experiencing the greatest limitations in functioning, with trip priority and complex booking systems creating overall inaccessibility.

Much of the literature on transportation for seniors is centred on the increasing number of older drivers. This has been interpreted to imply freedom, autonomy and flexibility (Ziegler and Schwanen, 2011), without considering that continued driving could be the result of a restrictive environment that does not accommodate alternative modes such as walking and public transit for the older population. Marottoli et al. (2000) found that for older adults, the cessation of driving was strongly associated with decreased activities outside the home. Without alternatives to the car, there are serious psychological implications when one must give up driving (Ragland et al., 2005). However, most research on aging and mobility is quantitative in nature and excludes an exploration of the meanings of immobility and unmet travel needs for older adults (Banister and Bowling, 2004).

Mobility is understood to be movement in physical space denoting the need for physical capacity and functioning. Intrinsic to the aging process is decline in functional capacity, though few authors have considered the impact on quality of life that this diminishing ability implies for mobility (Davey, 2007). While alternative transport such as para-transit may address the basic needs of seniors, trips for social connectedness and engagement that are imperative for well-being are not prioritized. Unmet mobility for the aging population has major implications for policy and planning, and, as the number of persons living past 80 years of age increases, greater understanding of the accessibility needs of this cohort will be essential to inform a transportation system that goes beyond traditional solutions (Alsnih and Hensher, 2003). To achieve inclusive mobility, a broader view of mobility and aging is necessary that seeks to address environmental and structural injustices.

Aging, mobility and the urban environment: an exclusionary view

Research on mobility considers transport "disadvantage" to occur when low rates of trip frequency are reported (Yigitcanlar et al., 2010). This definition is inadequate as a basis for understanding the existence of age-segregated environments that are characterized by inadequate access to transportation resources resulting from spatial, structural and material barriers (Gilroy, 2008). Generally, mobility has been regarded as a privilege rather than a right, which excludes older adults from normative methods of movement (Vannini, 2010). The aging population experiences mobility injustice primarily because of the unequal distribution of power and systematic obstacles to mobility, mobility options and access to space that create exclusionary processes (Kaufmann, 2002; Murray, 2015). To achieve social, economic and political equity, a more inclusive conceptualization of mobility for seniors is required.

The notion of motility is an overarching framework that reinforces the need for connectivity, service accessibility and community engagement to enhance healthy aging. Kaufmann's (2002) concept of motility is the capacity to be mobile; the nature of movement creates motility. Motility is unequally distributed as the result of hierarchies of power and, as such, is central to issues of sustainable mobility because this inequity creates social deprivation and exclusion (Stjernborg et al., 2014). Kaufmann (2002) identifies three constraints that limit movement and mobility including the capability of the person, the spatial environment, as well as systematic and structural barriers. It is notable that in the context of aging and mobility, personal capacity is overemphasized, while spatial factors and inequitable power relations are minimized (Murray, 2015).

The basis of mobility "justice" is effective and accessible transport. However, in the current urban context, there is a clear inequity based on access to automobile transportation (Yigitcanlar et al., 2010). Power is represented by a transportation infrastructure that enhances mobility for drivers, while entrenching social marginalization for those who lack this mobility resource (Dumbaugh, 2008). Key to the mobility injustice experienced by seniors is the ongoing change in the built environment resulting from a focus on automobile use and the spatial and policy dimensions of land-use patterns that support the predominance of a car-centric society.

In the early twentieth century, environments that included housing, services and social opportunities within the same neighborhood characterized urban design. The proximity of destinations enabled walking to be the main form of mobility, defining streets as places of commerce and communal assembly (Ladd, 2013). The original commercial and social uses of streets were subordinated, however, when the individual mobility of car travel began to dominate urban space in the 1950s. Fundamental changes in the social and economic order of society led to widespread automobile ownership, with the centralizing tendencies of walking being superseded by decentralized, auto-centred urban development.

Automobiles transformed cities, setting the agenda for urban and transportation planning. Urban infrastructure is now designed for "car culture" to facilitate vehicle flow, promote fast driving, acceleration and turns. Pedestrians are treated as obstructions to traffic effectively banning walking in these spaces (Ladd, 2013). The resulting environment has become car-oriented, out of human scale and characterized by prohibitive walking distances created by the separation of residential, industrial and commercial uses of the city (Lo, 2009). Nor can public transit services be offered efficiently or economically as city form has continued to spread. Cars have become a necessary aspect of urban life, but speed resulting in accidents and fatalities, emissions and health-threatening pollutants, use of space and traffic congestion also make them a fundamental urban problem (Ladd, 2013; Yigitcanlar et al., 2010).

To facilitate automobile travel, contemporary land-use patterns are based on monocentric development standards and practices, leading to urban sprawl and low-density suburban expansion (Yigitcanlar et al., 2010). Municipal guidelines encourage segregated land-use zones, low maximum densities, abundant free parking and cul-de-sac design of suburban development, promoting separation and exclusion of non-residents (Lo, 2009). The low-density design of urban space has resulted in systematic barriers and the mobility challenges faced by older adults is primarily the result of conventional community design practices. It is noteworthy, however, that in higher density communities with mixed land use offering a range of destinations, older adults use public transit and walk to destinations at much higher rates than those living in low-density environments (Dumbaugh, 2008).

The nominal response of city governments to address mobility injustice is to provide complex para-transit services that ultimately segregate those who cannot overcome the barriers of low-density development. A universal solution is needed to eliminate core barriers and integrate the mobility needs of all members of society within a single, inclusive framework (Dumbaugh, 2008). The foundation of such a community plan is based on innovative and sustainable principles to redesign the built environment and challenge traditional notions of community.

Age-inclusive places: an integrated vision of sustainability and mobility

A gerontological focus on urban design and planning has emerged only recently, initiated by the age-friendly movement that outlines elements of a neighborhood that are essential for creating places that support aging-in-place. The significance of this framework is its comprehensive view of accessibility and engagement, highlighting the linkage between transportation and social inclusion. Society overall, and the older population in particular, have become more aware of the significance of the built environment for healthy aging as a result. Nevertheless, the primary limitation of this concept is the lack of specific strategies on how age-friendly communities can be achieved. In moving forward, the creation of environments promoting both age inclusion and transportation accessibility requires a holistic and contextual approach that is embodied in the principles of urban sustainability.

With widespread concern about climate change, one of the most important global priorities currently is a sustainable urban future (Han et al., 2012). Urban sustainability proposes a paradigm that establishes the concurrent interaction of social, economic and environmental processes. These interactive domains identify planning innovations intended to create cities that are socially and economically equitable, as well as ecologically intact. Based on the synergies of these domains, sustainable mobility can be realized through spatial planning that incorporates higher density and mixed land-use development, the consolidation and reduction in distance of amenities and activities, and accessible transportation systems (Yigitcanlar, et al., 2010).

Urban sustainability highlights important mechanisms that could support older adults to remain in familiar community settings. However, the processes of aging have not been adequately incorporated into sustainable principles until now. Specifically, the impact of equity is not sufficiently integrated within the theory. This presents an opportunity to refine and align the social dimensions of sustainability with issues of quality of life, social justice and social cohesion that are paramount to maintaining a healthy aging population (Landorf et al., 2007). A more universal approach would promote design that accommodates all ranges of functioning and ability, improving the quality of life for older adults, while also improving environmental quality (Sykes and Robinson, 2014).

Though mobility is an important factor in both social equity and environmental transformation, current conceptions of sustainable transportation do not account for the marginalized and less mobile members of society. Transportation inequity is escalating in cities because of increasing distances to services and the inaccessibility of mobility resources. Policies should take into account social considerations, along with environmental and economic issues, and an individual's accessibility to urban opportunities that align with the social dimension of sustainability (Yigitcanlar et al., 2010).

Conceptualization of the principles of urban sustainability has generated a range of urban planning movements such as new urbanism, smart growth, compact cities and transit-oriented development. These emerging planning concepts propose strategies to reinvigorate communities and provide a meaningful alternative to urban sprawl. The basis of these strategies are guiding principles that promote accessible neighborhoods with mixed land uses, high-street connectivity and greater population density. Although they have rarely focused on distinct populations such as seniors (Michael et al., 2006), the goal of the proposed mobility-inclusive community plan is to balance the various dimensions of these approaches and highlight the potential for urban sustainability in support of aging-in-place.

Such strategies provide various design recommendations and planning directives to enable the transformation of existing neighborhoods that are responsive to an aging population. This examination of the potential of a mobility-inclusive community plan does not focus on one specific planning approach, but, rather, presents a range of concepts to illustrate the dynamics of place and the possibility of creating environments that enable aging-in-place. Instead of considering new urban development, this plan focuses on the redesign of existing communities where seniors are currently living.

The basic principle of urban sustainability is to reduce dependency on motor vehicles and diminish the need for excessive travel within cities. This can be achieved by urban planning policies that promote higher-density residential areas through community hubs of mixed use, simultaneously enhancing urban form that is pedestrian-friendly and that can support a comprehensive public transportation network. A more compact urban form based on integrated transport, infrastructure and services will more effectively respond to the needs of elderly people and adapt to an aging society (Han et al., 2012).

Mixed use

Mixed-used development is the cornerstone of sustainable urban design as it consolidates and intensifies the location of services, commercial retail and social and recreational opportunities. The premise of mixed-use development is to integrate a diverse and wide range of land uses and amenities so that a full range of activities are included in the community. Such development reduces the need to travel outside the residential neighborhood because of higher population densities. Less travel is required in mixed-use communities as there is a broadened ranged of services and social opportunities within the local environment.

As big retail outlets have replaced corner shops, distances to local activities have increased exponentially. To renew vibrancy in communities, the return of small grocery stores, banks, medical clinics, libraries, community and public services, and leisure and recreational centres is needed (Gilroy, 2008). These services and activities can be consolidated in the redevelopment of existing buildings, such as strip malls found along major streets that are surrounded by residential areas (Dumbaugh, 2008).

A further component of mixed-use space is the accommodation of a range of housing options within the neighborhood proximate to community service and recreational hubs. To promote aging-in-place, a variety of residential types can be offered, including single-detached homes in residential areas, as well as apartments and condominiums offering a continuum of services and levels of affordability. By accommodating individual needs and desires for housing, the area of mixed-use development will be enhanced with higher population density.

A crucial outcome of mixed-use design is the opportunity it provides to reduce automobile dependency, while advancing more sustainable forms of transportation (Yigitcanlar et al., 2010). Through higher densities, the redevelopment of spaces allows the creation of a multimodal transportation network that includes safe pedestrianism within the community, as well as a comprehensive transit system that enhances interconnectivity with linkages to various nodes of activity throughout the urban area.

Pedestrian facilities

Walkability is an important component of accessible and equitable sustainable communities (Lo, 2009). The presence of pedestrian-friendly design features, combined with mixed-use neighborhood centres, improves accessibility and minimizes the need for automobile travel. Until now, environmental interventions to encourage walking within neighborhoods have been based on the premise that increased walkability encourages physical activity and the promotion of health (Kerr et al., 2012). In contrast, the incorporation of pedestrianism in an urban sustainability plan is foundational for access to needed services and social opportunities within the local environment.

Developed pedestrian environments promote social interaction and enhance community cohesion. If desired destinations are one-quarter mile or less, walking is a viable mobility option for residents (Dunham-Jones, 2005). The literature (Hass-Klau, 2015; Lo, 2009; van Vliet, 2011) highlights several innovations to create walkable communities. To include pedestrians in regional planning processes, the following criteria should be included:

- A continuous and complete pedestrian network that mirrors the road network.
- Direct pedestrian routes with wide sidewalks and no obstacles.
- Safety through surveillance and activity.
- Protection from traffic, including crosswalks, traffic calming designs and reduced speed limits.
- The connectivity of pedestrian paths with street networks, transit service and other public spaces.
- Accessibility of facilities for people of all abilities that include places for resting.
- A stimulating environment that includes art, green spaces and planted flowers and trees.
- Good air quality, cleanliness and weather protection.

Public transportation

Effective public transportation balances its role as a node in a regional network with its provision of service within local areas (Dumbaugh, 2008). Along with a comprehensive pedestrian network, accessible and frequent public transportation routes are vital to access the mixed-use neighborhood centres of service and activities. Efficient and prompt transit services are also fundamental in the reduction of traffic congestion by offering a viable alternative to automobile use.

Ideally, a regional public transportation network should include some form of rail infrastructure that provides an off-road service that is not hindered by traffic congestion and that can serve expanding demand. In smaller metropolitan centres, such a system may not be economically feasible, but alternative options exist. A rapid transit line, for example, utilizes existing bus resources on a dedicated road, separated from congestion, with the flexibility to also share existing street space with vehicles.

There are several other considerations to designing an efficient public transportation system. First, it is crucial that sustainable public transit provide travel that is affordable. The location of public transportation should also be based on the main street routes of a community. To minimize mobility inequity, these transportation systems must incorporate routes that are comprehensive in spatial coverage and provide equal access to employment, housing, education, health services, commercial centres and recreation. A further element important for these systems is the accommodation of short-distance walks between place of residence and bus stops, as well as the connection to cycling and pedestrian systems (Yigitcanlar et al., 2010). When residential neighborhoods extend past one-quarter mile, shuttle services with regular schedules should be incorporated into the local environment to ensure similar access to main transit lines for all members of the community.

A mobility-inclusive community plan

The sustainable planning innovations of integrated neighborhoods that are pedestrian-oriented with mixed-use centres and comprehensive public transportation systems provide the basis to transform suburban areas into places supportive of enhanced quality of life. Fundamental is the human scale of mobility and service nodes that enable sustainable transportation within and between places of high-density, intergenerational living. Overall, the planning framework put forward strives to promote connectivity and pedestrian mobility, both essential to inclusive communities for aging.

Aging-in-place can be enriched by functional communities offering residential areas connected to centres of multiple land use that contain meaningful destinations accessible through pedestrian and transit corridors (Dumbaugh, 2008). This transformation of urban form substantiates the concept of a mobility-inclusive community plan. In the following section, I provide a case study to consider the feasibility of this proposal. The case study approach is important because, while there is an expansive literature advancing urban sustainability principles, it is more difficult to find examples of the implementation of these concepts in the context of city environments.

Case study: the potential for a place of inclusive mobility

The case study I chose to illustrate the potential application of the proposed mobility-inclusive community plan is Fort Garry, located in the south-central part of Winnipeg, Manitoba. This area was chosen as it contains the characteristics of an established inner suburb with a diverse population and an urban structure that has the potential to be redesigned into a sustainable community. This case study will demonstrate how a liveable environment based on mixed uses and alternative mobility options can be established.

Considered to be one of the oldest communities in Manitoba, Fort Garry originated with the development of the Pembina Trail, first used for the transport of furs and later as a route for new settlers traveling by oxcart from the south (Shipley, 1969). As the following discussion will demonstrate, it is significant that this trail lead to the historical Forks at the confluence of the Red and Assiniboine Rivers, now part of Winnipeg's downtown. In 1912, Fort Garry was incorporated into a municipality, joining the amalgamation of Winnipeg in 1972. The area is bounded by the Red River in the east, with the Jubilee overpass and St. Norbert defining its northern and southern extents and Waverley Street containing its western boundaries. The area of Fort Garry included in the case study is illustrated in Figure 1.1.

Fort Garry includes neighborhood elements to encourage sustainable mobility for all ages, thus ensuring the longevity of the older population to age-in-place. This urban setting provides a foundation to illustrate the vision of the mobility-inclusive community plan that proposes dense nodes of services and community activities overlaid with pedestrian and transit corridors. To expand upon this vision, the primary feature to emphasize is the arterial route of Pembina Highway that extends along the entire length of the community, providing a connecting link between the University of Manitoba and the central and downtown areas of Winnipeg. Pembina supplies the focus for the mobility-inclusive plan I am suggesting for Fort Garry.

Presently on Pembina Highway, there is constant car congestion as this heavily travelled main thoroughfare connects suburban commuters to the downtown and students to the university. It is also characterized by high residential density as the many apartment buildings along the street house both university students and an aging population seeking a more supportive living environment. As Figure 1.1 illustrates, there is a range of housing options for the senior population that is the basis for the application of the concept of centres of mixed use. Residential options include both a subsidized senior housing complex and an assisted living facility, as well as several naturally occurring retirement communities (NORCs), such as apartment blocks with a large concentration of older adults who have congregated there to age-in-place.

While the high population density situated on Pembina Highway should stimulate access to service opportunities, the street is typical of suburban development with an inhospitable pedestrian environment and scattered utilitarian strip malls offering mainly commercial outlets that are not consistent with the needs of the elderly. There is potential, nonetheless, given the high population density, to establish service-rich nodes with opportunities

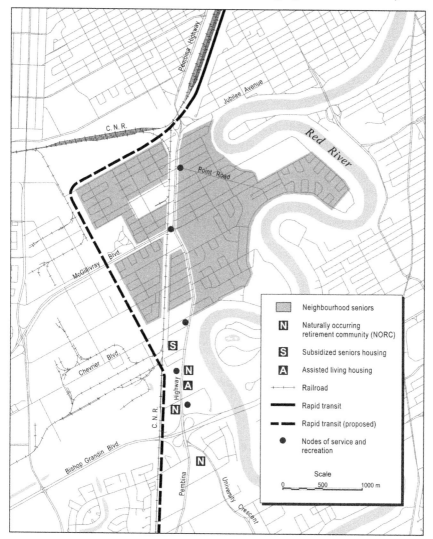

Figure 1.1 Fort Garry: a plan for a mobility-inclusive community

for socialization by implementing the mobility-inclusive community plan. In Figure 1.1, five such nodes are proposed that retrofit existing strip malls. These centres would provide local accessibility for both the older adults living on Pembina Highway, as well as seniors living in residential neighborhoods in the northern sections of Fort Garry.

Vital to the success of these central nodes of service and community cohesion would be a safe walking environment that provides connectivity between these centres and the apartment blocks where the older population resides. Such a pedestrian network would provide wide sidewalks with green space that accommodates resting stops. Paramount to the safety of older pedestrians in particular would be reduction of fast automobiles on Pembina Highway. However, the success of the five proposed community nodes focused on pedestrian accessibility will only occur with improvement in the public transportation network that encourages ridership and reduces traffic congestion.

There is currently a public transit route along Pembina Highway utilized mainly to transport university students. This bus network is connected to the first phase of a rapid transit line originating in the downtown area. The route currently runs at maximum capacity and provides limited access for older adults living in Fort Garry, as full buses with few available seats run between the downtown and the university campus throughout the day. A more efficient network system is necessary that incorporates the needs of all potential users.

Previously, there was potential for improved service as the City of Winnipeg originally planned to extend the rapid transit line along the rail tracks that are parallel to Pembina Highway. Public transportation would have become feasible for older residents along the main artery, accommodating an increased number of buses with safer and more comfortable service. The pedestrian network could have been extended to the new rapid transit line and those living in more distant neighborhoods could have been connected through local shuttle services. However, the city government made the controversial decision to route the new line further west along Waverley Street, failing to embrace an opportunity to create connectivity to the city as a whole for the existing community population of Fort Garry. This demonstrates the many barriers that exist within current structures and society to promote an age-friendly environment.

If the mobility-inclusive plan was implemented in Fort Garry to include the rapid transit line, these sustainable planning principles could reinvigorate the community and provide a meaningful alternative to continuing urban sprawl. By accommodating and integrating a diverse and wide range of land uses and providing accessibility to community nodes through comprehensive pedestrian and public transit corridors, there would be greater service and social opportunities for the older population supporting the primary objective of the plan for aging-in-place. A vibrant community would also encourage increased population density and housing choices, allowing for further development of vacant land in Fort Garry and thereby exemplifying the value of urban sustainability for a healthier community overall.

Conclusion: achieving age-inclusive mobility

The case study of Fort Garry reveals a plan for integrated community design that promotes inclusive-mobility and creates social equity for all community members. The plan I have proposed is based on the concept of urban sustainability illustrating that the integration of social, economic and environmental goals can promote places that are supportive for aging-in-place. The foundation of this plan is the establishment of a comprehensive pedestrian and public transportation infrastructure that provides accessibility to mixed-use centres of service and social opportunities, promoting higher-density living without reliance on automobile use.

The general assumption is that it is too difficult to change the built environment. By illustrating the feasibility of connecting aging-in-place to urban sustainability, society will begin to recognize its benefits and viability. The application of the proposed mobility-inclusive community plan underscores the potential for retrofitting existing suburbs and promoting aging-in-place. It also provides a baseline for the design and planning of new developments that are age-integrated.

Spaces have traditionally been designed from a top-down approach of powerful planning mechanisms. More effective are strategies that raise awareness of unsustainable transportation patterns and that seek community collaboration on development decisions (Yigitcanlar et al., 2010). Programs can be developed, for example, to empower older adults in advocating for changes in zoning codes and regulations regarding the built environment (Sykes and Robinson, 2014). There is a need for a flexible and adaptive environment according to the changing abilities, desires and needs of residents (Antoninetti and Garrett, 2012).

Investigative research with seniors is needed to further examine the impact of unmet mobility needs, while also consulting with them regarding the characteristics of their neighborhoods and the perceived qualities that are essential to allow them to age-in-place. Such knowledge will be essential to further expand the mobility-inclusive community framework proposed in this chapter. Further examination is also required of communities that presently portray good design practices of mixed uses that offer social cohesion through safe pedestrian environments, effective public transit and a range of housing options.

The discourse on inclusive mobility and urban sustainability has demonstrated that design practices to reclaim urban space for pedestrians, and to establish alternative modes of transit while promoting community cohesion, are a valuable enterprise to support independent living for the aging population (Gilroy, 2008; Ladd, 2013). The proposal of a mobility-inclusive community plan represents a first step in integrating the needs of an aging population with the universal goals of environmental sustainability, social equity and economic viability.

References

Alsnih, R. and Hensher, D.A. (2003). The mobility and accessibility expectations of seniors in an aging population. *Transportation Research Part A: Policy and Practice*, 37(10), 903–916.

Antoninetti, M. and Garrett, M. (2012). Body capital and the geography of aging. *Area*, *44*(3), 364–370.

Banister, D. and Bowling, A. (2004). Quality of life for the elderly: The transport dimension. *Transport Policy*, *11*(2), 105–115.

Davey, J.A. (2007). Older people and transport: Coping without a car. *Aging and Society*, *27*(1), 49–65.

Dumbaugh, E. (2008). Designing communities to enhance the safety and mobility of older adults. *Journal of Planning Literature*, *23*(1), 17–36.

Dunham-Jones, E. (2005). Suburban retrofits, demographics, and sustainability. *Places*, *17*(2), 8–19.

Fobker, S. and Grotz, R. (2006). Everyday mobility of elderly people in different urban settings: The example of the city of Bonn, Germany. *Urban Studies*, *43*(1), 99–118.

Gilroy, R. (2008). Places that support human flourishing: Lessons from later life. *Planning Theory & Practice*, *9*(2), 145–163.

Han, J., Fontanos, P., Fukushi, K., Herath, S., Heeren, N., Naso, V., Cecchi, C., Edwards, P. and Takeuchi, K. (2012). Innovation for sustainability: Toward a sustainable urban future in industrialized cities. *Sustainability Science*, *7*(1), 91–100.

Hass-Klau, C. (2015). *The Pedestrian and the City*. New York: Routledge.

Kaufmann, V. (2002). *Rethinking Mobility: Contemporary Sociology*. Ashgate: Aldershot.

Kerr, J., Rosenberg, D. and Frank, L. (2012). The role of the built environment in healthy ageing: Community design, physical activity and health among older adults. *Journal of Planning Literature*, *27*(1), 43–60.

Ladd, B. (2013). Cities on wheels: Cars and public space. In G. Bridge and S. Watson (eds), *The New Blackwell Companion to the City*, 265–274. Toronto, ON: Wiley Blackwell.

Landorf, C., Brewer, G. and Sheppard, L. (2007). Urban sustainability and ageing: Uncovering the critical links between the urban environment and successful ageing in place. In M. Horner, C. Hardcastle, A. Price and J. Bebbington (eds), 27–29 June 2007, *International Conference on Whole Life Urban Sustainability and its Assessment*.Glasgow.

Lo, R.H. (2009). Walkability: What is it? *Journal of Urbanism*, *2*(2), 145–166.

Marottoli, R.A., de Leon, C.F.M., Glass, T.A., Williams, C.S., Cooney, L.M. and Berkman, L.F. (2000). Consequences of driving cessation decreased out-of-home activity levels. *Journals of Gerontology, Series B: Psychological Sciences and Social Sciences*, *55*(6), S334–S340.

Metz, D.H. (2000). Mobility of older people and their quality of life. *Transport Policy*, *7*(2), 149–152.

Michael, Y.L., Green, M.K. and Farquhar, A. (2006). Neighbourhood design and active aging. *Health & Place*, *12*, 734–740.

Murray, L. (2015). Age-friendly mobilities: A transdisciplinary and intergenerational perspective. *Journal of Transport & Health*, *2*, 302–307.

Paez, A., Scott, D., Potoglou, D., Kanaroglou, P. and Newbold, K.B. (2007). Elderly mobility: Demographic and spatial analysis of trip making in the Hamilton CMA, Canada. *Urban Studies*, *44*(1), 123–146.

Ragland, D.R., Satariano, W.A. and MacLeod, K.E. (2005). Driving cessation and increased depressive symptoms. *Journals of Gerontology, Series A: Biological Sciences and Medical Sciences*, *60*(3), 399–403.

Schwanen, T., Banister, D. and Bowling, A. (2012). Independence and mobility in later life. *Geoforum, 43*(6), 1313–1322.

Shipley, N. (1969). *Road to the Forks: A History of the Community of Fort Garry.* Winnipeg, MB: Stovel Advocate Press.

Spinney, J.E., Scott, D.M. and Newbold, K.B. (2009). Transport mobility benefits and quality of life: A time-use perspective of elderly Canadians. *Transport Policy, 16*(1), 1–11.

Stjernborg, V., Wretstrand, A. and Tesfahuney, M. (2014). Everyday life mobilities of older persons: A case study of ageing in a suburban landscape in Sweden. *Mobilities, 10*(3), 383–401.

Sykes, K.E. and Robinson, K.N. (2014). Making the right moves: Promoting smart growth and active aging in communities. *Journal of Aging & Social Policy, 26*, 166–180.

van Vliet, W. (2011). Intergenerational cities: A framework for policies and programs. *Journal of Intergenerational Relationships, 9*, 348–365.

Vannini, P. (2010). Mobile cultures: From the sociology of transportation to the study of mobilities. *Sociology Compass, 4*(2), 111–121.

Yigitcanlar, T., Rashid, K. and Dur, F. (2010). Sustainable urban and transport development for transportation disadvantaged: A review. *The Open Transportation Journal, 4*, 1–8.

Ziegler, F. and Schwanen, T. (2011). "I like to go out to be energised by different people": An exploratory analysis of mobility and wellbeing in later life. *Aging and Society, 31*(5), 758–781.

2 Portrayal of older adults in popular television shows

Margaret Waltz and Brian K. Gran

As people grow older, their identities change (Sneed and Whitbourne, 2005). Likewise, as populations age, how older people are depicted in mass media changes. This chapter examines how popular television shows depict older people. Its approach is comparative. We examine five TV shows popular in Canada, the United Kingdom (UK) and the United States (US).

Sociologists have paid attention to *identity* as a feature of social interaction. George Herbert Mead (1934) said that community and autonomy are necessary ingredients of identity, while Erving Goffman advanced different notions of identity. Goffman's idea of "personal identity" is a set of traits and characteristics that make a person an individual in other people's minds (Goffman, 1963; Branaman, 1997). His notion of "self-identity" is a person's own awareness of her situation and its relationship to her background and character (Goffman, 1963; Branaman, 1997). A third identity, according to Goffman, is "social identity," which is a person's identifying factors from another person's perspective, such as the individual's age and gender (Jenkins, 2014).

A perspective on identity noted by Andriot and Owens (2012) intersects with Mead and Goffman's ideas. This perspective identifies personal identity, role identity, social identity and collective identity. Personal identity arises from an amalgam of a person's biography, her own characteristics, role identities and experiences. In contrast, role identity is the role a person plays in a position when interacting within a group. A person's social identity is from social interaction and where and how a person fits into a group. Collective identity is when individuals' interaction as a group leads to a shared identity.

Given that sociologists view identity as socially constructed, it follows that identity will continue to change over individuals' life courses. An older individual's personal identity will continue to change according to her/his unique history. Similarly, self-identity will continue to change because an individual's situation, history and character will continue to change. An older individual's social identity may come to reflect external changes many people associate with aging, including wrinkles and grey hair.

Media are means of communication, whether through print, digital or audiovisual. Anything from a poster to an article online to a video game to an independent or major motion picture are forms of media. Mass media is defined as a medium that reaches a wide audience, or a mass of people. But as Mills (1956) suggests, very few individuals or organizations are able to reach this mass and to disseminate their ideas widely. This point intersects with Marx's (1932, p. 655) theory of historical materialism, that "the ideas of the ruling class are in every epoch the ruling ideas." Because those with power have a greater ability to distribute and communicate ideas en masse, they also have the ability to shape the ideas of those who consume media, intentionally or not. Currently in the US, for instance, six corporations own and construct 90 percent of US media (Lutz, 2012).

Mass media matters to identity construction because it works as an agent of socialization, shaping the values, norms and ideas of people who consume it—and they consume a lot of it. For instance, people living in Canada and the UK watch an average of 28–30 hours of television per week (BBC News, 2013; Television Bureau of Canada, 2015), while people in the US watch an average of 35 hours of TV each week (Bureau of Labor Statistics, 2015). Because so few individuals and groups have control over the mass media that people consume, a very narrow range of values, norms and ideas are presented, which leads to the development and perpetuation of stereotypes. These stereotypes, and portrayals of characters and groups more generally, influence people's perceptions of social groups as well as what people think about themselves and their place in society.

Given that many components of mass media serve to perpetuate stereotypes and to influence the identities of many groups, including women and people of color, why care about mass media's construction of "older adult" identities? While there has been an increase in the number of older characters in mass media in recent decades, older adults, especially older women, are still rarely portrayed, rendering them largely invisible on TV and in other forms of mass media (Vernon et al., 1990; Vickers, 2007). When older adults are represented, research has shown that they have been portrayed as ugly, senile, ill, one dimensional, less friendly and less sexually active than younger characters, with older women more negatively portrayed than men (Vernon et al., 1990; Bazzini et al., 1997). In stark contrast, older adults can also be presented as "super seniors" who are healthy, wealthy and basically age defying—distorting reality and "reflecting the dominance of independence, youthfulness, effectiveness, and productivity as values in Western societies" (Milner et al., 2011, p. 27). Given their relative invisibility on TV, these representations of older adults that do exist are all the more meaningful. In fact, portrayals of aging have not only been shown to negatively impact older people's self-perceptions, self-esteem and self-efficacy, they also have been shown to negatively impact their health (Milner et al., 2011). It is, therefore, important to understand how older adults are portrayed in popular TV shows and whether these portrayals of older adults vary across cultures that have a global TV presence.

Comparative approach and case selection

Our approach to the study can be broken down as a series of steps. First, we focused on contemporary shows to ensure that this was a comparison of television shows that have been broadcast in the same period. This approach minimizes differences in shows that are in response to external events and circumstances. However, one might ask, why compare television shows from Canada, the UK and the US? Beyond the ease of analyzing television shows broadcast in our own language, which is English, we selected these three countries because of their similarities and differences. When comparing Canada, the UK and the US, it is often assumed that they have many similarities. For instance, in his groundbreaking work on welfare states, Esping-Andersen (1990, 1999) asserts that these three countries are liberal welfare regimes. Liberal welfare regimes are characterized as relying on markets to produce and distribute social goods. According to the liberal typology, people living in these countries are expected to be self-reliant, rather than relying on government to succeed.

Of course, Canada, the UK and the US have backgrounds that flow from their shared cultural, economic, political and social histories. While various languages are spoken in each country, English is one of the key languages spoken in all three countries. All three countries are considered western democracies sharing similar governmental and legal systems. The histories of Canada and the US are inextricably tied to the UK, given that Canada is a Commonwealth country and the US is a former British colony.

Yet, anyone who has lived in Canada, the UK or the US can tell you these three countries are significantly different in many respects. From cultural attitudes to socio-political structures, including their welfare states (Gran 2008), people living in these countries can have different experiences. Canada and the US have among the most diverse populations in the world. Even popular sports tend to differ, from hockey in Canada to soccer (called football in the UK) to American football (not soccer). Most Canadian and UK residents enjoy universal health insurance coverage and US residents have health insurance coverage from a "hodge podge" of sources, from public to private to public–private mixes.

One aspect of each country that is roughly similar is the proportion of the population aged 65 and older. For Canada, this proportion was 15.72 percent in 2014; for the UK it was 16.98 percent for 2013 and for the US the proportion was 14.5 percent for 2014 (OECD, 2014). Given that the proportion of older people aged 65 and older for Organisation for Economic Co-operation and Development (OECD) countries ranges from 25.06 percent (Japan) to 6.5 percent (Mexico), Canada, the UK and the US lie in the middle of their OECD peers (OECD, 2014).

Our first step in the research process was to ask the question: how are aging and elderly people depicted in popular television shows? Our second step was to identify what television shows to watch from across the selected countries, and we chose to examine five popular TV shows in total. These included *Blackstone* (Canada) (Scott, 2011), *Grace and Frankie* (US) (Kauffman et al., 2015a), *Downton Abbey* (UK) (Fellowes et al., 2011), *Last Tango in Halifax* (UK) (Shindler, 2012) and *Parenthood* (US) (Howard et al., 2013). Each television show has aired in the past five years and features prominent characters who are older adults. The shows have also been renewed for more than one season and all five shows have received or have been nominated for prominent awards—which was taken to be an indicator of popularity. *Downton Abbey* won Golden Globe, Emmy and BAFTA awards. *Parenthood* has been nominated for Golden Globe and Critics' Choice awards. *Blackstone* has won multiple Gemini, Leo and Canadian Screen awards. *Last Tango in Halifax* has won a BAFTA award for the series and multiple nominations for acting. The newest series, *Grace and Frankie*, has won an OFTA award and received Golden Globe and Emmy nominations.

We watched all episodes of each series. Our goal was not only to focus on specific episodes, but to comprehend characterizations and relationships, changes in characterizations and relationships and references to social worlds outside the television series. For instance, the television show, *Blackstone*, refers to the socio-politics surrounding First Nations of Canada.

After identifying and observing the TV shows, our third step was to employ a content analysis of what we watched. A benefit of employing content analysis in this study is the ability to examine a television show holistically. Rather than focussing on a single character or episode, content analysis enabled us to study characters, their trajectories and their relationships over seasons (or season, in the case of *Grace and Frankie*). In this way, we employed a more ethnographic content analysis as opposed to a more quantitative content analysis (Altheide, 1987).

The term "character arc" refers to the changes a character experiences in her/his personality from the beginning of a series through events that unfold around and to the character up to the end of the story. Gradually she/he changes in what is described as an "arc" that is complete when the story is over (Bell, 2004). Thus, content analysis empowered us to study the "arc" of a character as well as relationships between characters. Using established practices associated with content analysis, we identified topics and themes central to each television show. An important topic of *Grace and Frankie*, for example, was significant, surprising changes in relationships and their consequences for the individuals in those relationships and individuals tied to those relationships. After the husbands of Grace and Frankie reveal that they are gay and in love, a great deal of the content of this television show is devoted to how these two revelations change the lives of people surrounding the husbands. We paid attention to which characters played prominent roles in the television show and attempted to discern reasons for this. For example, a character in *Blackstone* is filming a documentary and he plays multiple roles, from collecting perspectives of the community's history to investigations of corruption and failure. This character represents a person communicating information about and from the community to outsiders, including viewers.

The depiction of older adults in TV shows in Canada, the UK and the US revolves around three similar themes which we discuss below: later life as a period of transition, older adults as wise and older adults challenging political authority.

Findings

Later-life transitions

The first theme that we identified is that later life can serve as a period of transition. Older characters in the shows chosen from the UK and the US are portrayed as going through or preparing to go through major life changes. The US show *Parenthood*, for example, features the characters Camille and Zeek who are in their late 60s to early 70s. In Season 5, Episode 2, these characters disagree over whether to downsize from their large house to a condo (Hudgins and Trilling, 2013). Camille wants to move to a condo for the opportunity to live near museums and restaurants. She also wants to travel and living in a condo would provide the money to do so and to start their "act three," their last big finale in life, while they are still young enough to enjoy these opportunities (Hudgins and Trilling, 2013). In Season 5, Episode 3, Zeek does not want to leave his house, citing it as a place full of memories that he does not want to leave. He also says that he has traveled and he does not like any place else, crushing Camille who says she has never left the country and feels she has lost her voice in their marriage (Watson and Norris, 2013).

While the portrayal of Zeek plays into the stereotype of a sort of "stick in the mud" older character, grumpy and resistant to change, Camille breaks the mold of traditional portrayals of older characters. She reflects upon her unhappiness and the lack of opportunities she has had in her marriage and as a stay-at-home mom throughout most of her life. She now seeks an identity change. Her age and position in the life course has provided her with the ability to create that change because her children are grown and out of the house. She therefore takes a risk and decides to travel to Italy for a month with her art class and tells Zeek that she is going without him. Camille finds independence and begins her "third act"—to fulfill needs that have gone unmet in her life so far. This action sways Zeek to pursue a "third act" with Camille and to downsize to a condo upon her return.

The UK television show *Last Tango in Halifax* depicts a later-life transition more in line with the one presented in *Parenthood* than *Grace and Frankie*. *Last Tango in Halifax* centres around Celia and Alan, both of whom are in their 70s and widowed. They were schoolmates that had not seen each other since 1953. They were interested in each other then, but after a series of unfortunate events, they married other people. They meet again after reconnecting on Facebook and reflect on their marriages (Wainwright and Lyn, 2012a). Celia describes how her husband cheated on her and that she has felt unhappy for the past 40 years. Alan describes how his wife died of Alzheimer's and did not know him at the end of her life. While he was content with his wife, he says that Celia is and always was his true love. By the end of the first episode, they decide to get married, finding another chance at happiness that they missed out on in their youth and middle age (Wainwright and Lyn, 2012a). There is also a sense that they do not want to waste time, not because there is not necessarily a lot of time left in their lives, but because of what was lost and what "could have been" in the past.

Much like Camille in *Parenthood*, Celia and Alan enact this transition late in their lives in order to seek the happiness that escaped them in their pasts. This transition brings them joy, illustrating that later life holds opportunities and possibilities for their characters, unlike stereotypical representations of older adults and later life that suggest old age is boring, routine and without new opportunities. But while this transition sparks positive change for Celia and Alan, Season 1 shows that it is more difficult for their children to handle. Celia and Alan each have one daughter and neither daughter is particularly comfortable with their respective parent's engagement, not because of the parent's age, but because it is perceived that this engagement reshapes family history (Wainwright and Lyn, 2012b). The daughters have difficulty acknowledging that their parents were not happy with their spouses and longed to be with other people for most of their lives. This diminishes the daughters' perceptions of their late parents. Celia's daughter Caroline even questions whether Celia wishes she could go back in time and marry Alan instead, meaning that Caroline would have never been born. As the matriarch and patriarch of their respective families, Celia and Alan's later-life transition creates change for the rest of their families as well.

A central theme of *Grace and Frankie* is also later-life transition. In this recently launched series, two major later-life transitions are the basis of its comedy and drama. Two heterosexual couples have been friends for decades, with their husbands working as partners in a domestic relations (e.g., divorce) law firm. When same-sex marriage is legalized, the husbands reveal to their wives that they are gay, in love and plan to marry after they divorce their wives (Kauffman et al., 2015b). Unstated, but implicit, is that the husbands would have continued their hidden affair if same-sex marriage had not become legal. Ending their heterosexual marriages and taking steps to form their same-sex marriage is one of Grace and Frankie's significant life transitions.

The second theme of *Grace and Frankie* is the wives' realizations that their marriages to their husbands have been charades (Kauffman et al., 2015b). As Grace, played by well-known actress Jane Fonda, looks around her husband's at-home study, she discovers homo-erotic art and artifacts to which she has turned a "blind eye" for years. Frankie, played by equally well known actress Lily Tomlin, is broken hearted. Frankie seems to still love her husband, Sol, who is played by Sam Watterson. While Grace's concerns seem to focus on material possessions, such as who will own which house, Frankie is more struck by the loss of her marriage to Sol.

Overall, this theme contrasts from usual portrayals of older adults as one dimensional, sexually inactive, senile, or ill (Vernon et al., 1990; Bazzini et al., 1997). This is especially true in *Parenthood* and *Last Tango in Halifax* as the characters in both of these shows are actively thinking about their "third act." These "third acts" are presented by the writers as full of possibility and as having the potential to be better than, or at least equivalent to, the first two "acts" of younger life.

Wise old men and women

The second theme that we identified in our viewing is that older characters in the TV shows from Canada, the UK and the US are portrayed as wise old men and women, but they also challenge this classic archetype. In the Canadian show *Blackstone*, for instance, the character Cecil Delaronde is presented as a wise old man. In an early scene of Season 1, Episode 1, Delaronde is being interviewed and filmed as he talks about Native culture, in particular, "the Creation story" (Cardinal and Scott, 2011). As the transition is made from a scene of young people getting high on illicit drugs to Delaronde, we hear Delaronde discuss this story of the "Creator" who is sending out his thoughts to people and waiting for those thoughts to return. *Blackstone*'s writing team is trying to communicate to viewers that Native Canadians are using drugs to turn off their minds so they do not hear their Creator. When the interviewer, Victor Merasty, played by actor Nathaniel Arcand, takes down the video equipment, Delaronde continues to talk about Native culture. According to Delaronde, culture is

> the old days, the old ways, the good stuff that makes us who we are. But it's also what goes on today. If you look around you, culture is on display every day. Family violence. Alcoholism. Drug abuse. Incest. Suicide. Corruption. That's our culture now.
>
> (Cardinal and Scott, 2011)

It is clear that the show's writers treat Delaronde as a person who possesses authority because his roots are shown to be part of the past, not of the present. The past is depicted as a time without corruption, without self-harm of alcohol abuse and illegal drug abuse, without family violence and other harmful things. It is a time of purity from the past when Native people did not hurt themselves and each other. The present is a time of corruption and violence. Delaronde has moral authority because he does not take part in contemporary corruption and violence.

Later, when a Chief is to be elected, Delaronde speaks up for a new Chief, not the incumbent, calling for change. He uses his moral authority to bolster the campaign of the candidate as well as to give hope to the band. This candidate, Leona Stoney, played by actress Carmen Moore, wins the election. The incumbent Chief, Andy Fraser, played by Native Canadian Eric Schweig, storms out and lashes out at everyone, including Stoney, Merasty and Delaronde, describing them with derogatory racist expletives (Cardinal and Scott, 2011).

In *Downton Abbey*, Maggie Smith plays Violet Crawley, the Dowager Countess and matriarch of the Crawley family, and she symbolizes tradition and the "old world." While the series starts in 1912, Violet still dresses in traditional Victorian style, complete with a bustle. She is also hesitant to accept change, even expressing her dislike for the glare and vapors produced by electricity, as it makes her feel like she is "on stage at the Gaiety." Much like Delaronde's character, Violet has traditional authority within her family and the town of Downton. For example, in Season 1, Episode 2, when her American daughter-in-law, Cora, suggests to Violet's granddaughter, Mary, that Mary pursue and marry the new heir to the Crawley fortune, Mary rebukes the idea saying that her American mother does not understand English ways (Fellowes and Bolt, 2010). When Cora tells Mary that the marriage was Violet's idea, Mary is shocked and takes the suggestion more seriously, illustrating how Violet is seen as a wise old woman who is aware of, and has authority over, the customs and protocols of social life. What makes the representation of Violet different than that of other archetypal wise and old figures is that she is portrayed as being "wise" and rooted in tradition through her wit, giving her charisma as well as authority. While she is the "comic relief" in the series, the humor stems from the profound nature of what she says, not because she is out of touch, senile or one dimensional, as older adults are often portrayed.

The show *Grace and Frankie* challenges the conception of older characters as wise stalwarts of tradition. After learning their husbands are leaving them for each other, in Season 1, Episode 1, Grace and Frankie each turn to mind-altering substances (Kauffman et al., 2015b). Grace regularly copes by consuming alcohol and pharmaceutical prescriptions. The day after learning her husband, Robert, played by Martin Sheen, is leaving her for Sol, Frankie's husband, Grace's daughters come to their family home. After learning of the news, they console their mother by getting her two valium pills (and ones for themselves). Grace eventually travels to a beach house that the two couples jointly own. She tells Robert that he can have the house, but she wants him to buy out Frankie and Sol from the beach house, then give the beach house to her.

Frankie is depicted as a former hippie in the clothes she wears and how she behaves. Grace even calls her "hippie dippie." After visiting a liquor store to buy junk food and booze, Frankie also travels to the beach house where she turns to meditation and consumes peyote, a hallucinogen found in Mexico and Texas and associated with Native American culture (Kauffman et al., 2015b). Later that evening, as she sits by a fire on the beach, Frankie chants and plays a musical instrument. She experiences a back spasm and Grace brings Frankie's muscle relaxants to her. As they both consume Frankie's prescription, Grace takes a drink from Frankie's "tea," which is the peyote. They stay up all night, dancing, chanting and consoling each other on the beach. Their peyote experience produces insights and wisdom about their marriages, families and their futures (Kauffman et al., 2015b).

A common aspect that runs through all of these shows is how they characterize wisdom. To be wise requires turning to and valuing insights from the past. In *Blackstone* and *Downton Abbey*, older characters draw upon past cultural practices that members of their contemporary societies ignore or, worse, belittle. To gain wisdom, Grace and Frankie turn to mind-altering substances associated with hippies and Native American cultures.

Historical locations

The final theme that we identified in our viewing is that the lives of older characters in TV shows from Canada, the UK and the US are shaped by their historical locations. In *Grace and Frankie*, for example, an overarching theme is how same-sex marriage in the US matters to everyone and can change everyone's lives. Robert and Sol have managed an affair behind their wives' backs for 20 years. "Because we can" is the primary reason Robert and Sol give for ending their marriages *now* and marrying each other *now* (Kauffman et al., 2015b). In their bid to be "truly" happy, Robert and Sol end their heterosexual marriages and disrupt their families' lives. The adult children of Grace and the adult children of Frankie are initially shocked and express outrage when they learn of their fathers' decisions to divorce their mothers and to marry each other. Grace has two daughters, Mallory, played by Brooklyn Decker, and Brianna, played by June Diane Raphael. After hearing the news of her parents' divorce and her father's relationship with Sol, Mallory rhetorically asks what she will tell her kids? Robert seems speechless.

Both Grace and Frankie express outrage at having invested years of energy and time, as well as having given up opportunities to support their husbands' careers and marriages. As noted above, now that their children are adults and their husbands' careers are concluding, Grace and Frankie had been looking forward to the "third acts" of their marriages and lives. In a scene in Season 1, Episode 1 where Frankie and Grace are sitting by a fire on the beach, Grace looks up to the sky and rages:

> I did everything right, Lord. I stood by him for over 40 years. I raised his children. I shopped with his mother. I did every single thing so he wouldn't have to worry about it. I played by all of the rules. Why didn't you tell me there were no rules? It's not fair.
>
> (Kauffman et al., 2015b)

These statements could apply to any divorce, of course, but have special resonance for Grace and Frankie. Not only were Grace and Frankie looking forward to spending retirement with their husbands, they were planning to stay married to their husbands until death. Grace's soliloquy to God expresses frustration that there are "no rules." However, one "rule" that has produced significant change in the lives of the couples and their children is legalization of same-sex marriage. Without this change, Grace and Frankie may have performed their "third act" as they had planned. Instead, this change in US law has changed the lives of these and many other families across the US. Grace probably is wrong about rules; rather than "no rules," we have new rules.

In *Downton Abbey*, Violet Crawley's life is also influenced by her historical location. As previously stated, the story begins in 1912 and the two closest heirs to the Crawley estate and title have died on the ship Titanic. In Series 1, Episode 1, another relation, a third cousin once removed, is introduced and, unknown to the family, this cousin will soon inherit the title and the family's money instead of Violet's granddaughter (Fellowes and Percival, 2010). This is because, by UK law in this time period, a woman did not have inheritance rights. Before suggesting that her granddaughter, Mary, engage in wedlock with the new heir to keep the money in the family, Violet does everything in her power to "break the entail," or, in other words, to dispute the law about inheritance to ensure that the family's money and estate go to Mary. While there is no way for Mary to inherit the title, breaking the entail would at least maintain the family's authority over Downton. As Violet says, "I didn't run Downton for 30 years to see it go lock, stock, and barrel to a stranger from God knows where" (Fellowes and Percival, 2010). Violet's historical and social location initially gave her status, money and power, but, at the same time, the laws of the time threaten all that she and her family have worked for.

A key theme of *Blackstone* is the breakdown and corruption of contemporary society in this Native Canadian band/community. As noted, the series' writers enable characters' experiences from contemporary society to contrast with recollections of the past. In the past, the band and its members relied on Native traditions to function and govern. In contrast, now the band's leaders are corrupt. The band is afflicted with violence and corruption. *Blackstone* depicts the Chief and his aides as abusing their leadership positions of trust. When, during a band meeting, a younger member asks for results of the band's financial audit, the political leaders chide the young man for not understanding how the band works and for failing to appreciate their leadership (Cardinal and Scott, 2011). Delaronde, the wise older member, stands up for the young member. Delaronde insists that this young man, as a band member, has a right to this information just the same as any other band member. The political leaders do not challenge Delaronde, who represents purity of past cultural practices.

A common aspect of these shows is how the characters' historical locations influence their lives. In *Grace and Frankie* and *Downton Abbey*, older characters' lives and choices are subject to the laws of the time, both new laws reflecting social change and old laws that are beginning to seem outdated. In the background of *Blackstone* is significant legal change affecting relations between First Nations and the Canadian government. In the context of the community of *Blackstone*, there is an awareness of the change that has occurred in the band over time. On the one hand, the band has moved away from its traditional ways. On the other hand, the band is struggling to form its new identity as its members seek to overcome manifold social problems, from substance abuse to family breakdown to violence and corruption. Delaronde is the key character who not only maintains an awareness of past traditions and ways, but also a willingness to speak up and challenge the band as it travels in what he and others consider to be the wrong direction.

Conclusion

There were three themes that were identified in our viewing of *Blackstone*, *Downton Abbey*, *Grace and Frankie*, *Last Tango in Halifax* and *Parenthood*. First, older adulthood serves as a period of transition, a "third act" that is presented as full of possibility and as having the potential for a happiness that the characters may have missed out on earlier in life. Second, older adults are characterized as wise, enacting the archetype of the "wise old man" or "wise old woman." However, these TV shows also challenge this representation, portraying older characters as witty or striving to gain the wisdom that they lack. Finally, the historical locations where older characters' live, work, raise families and form communities greatly influence their choices and abilities in both restrictive and permissive ways.

Our methodological approach was to compare television shows originally broadcast in three countries: Canada, the UK and the US. Taking J.S. Mill's (1956) methods as our starting point, we selected these three countries because of their similarities, such as their historical, political and social ties. Another similarity is the proportion of their populations that are age 65 and older, which ranges from 14.5 percent to nearly 17 percent. This similarity provides confidence that the television shows are not responding to heightened concerns about large older populations, or do not include older characters because the country's older population is small. At the same time, we recognize that differences exist between these countries. These differences may shape what television shows are broadcast and what their content is. From these similarities and differences emerge the themes of the third act, wisdom and historical location. These portrayals of older adults challenge traditional conceptions and depictions of older adulthood in popular television as one dimensional—a time in people's lives that is often depicted as involving senility, illness or sexual inactivity.

However, these older characters are representative of a very limited number of social groups. For instance, with the exception of *Blackstone*, these shows portray little racial or ethnic diversity. Despite an adopted African American son on *Grace and Frankie* and an African American daughter-in-law and mixed-race grandson on *Parenthood*, the primary characters on *Grace and Frankie* and *Parenthood* and all of the characters on *Last Tango in Halifax* and *Downton Abbey* are white. Moreover, all of the older characters on these four shows are also white. As a result, these four shows fail to offer diverse portrayals of older characters in terms of race and ethnicity.

The same is true of social class. The older characters in *Grace and Frankie*, *Downton Abbey*, *Last Tango in Halifax* and *Parenthood* are all of high social class standing. They face very few money troubles and are able to retire from, if they ever worked in, the paid labour market. Yet, many of the problems these older characters face are a result of their wealth. For instance, Camille and Zeek would not face the question of whether to move to a condo in the cultural centre of San Francisco, and Camille could not have found her independence and taken her trip to Italy, without financial resources. An issue for the two couples at the centre of *Grace and Frankie* is that they must divide assets during their divorces. These assets include multiple homes, including a house on the ocean.

Blackstone is distinct from the other four shows in its focus on Native Canadians. When a non-Native Canadian character appears on *Blackstone*, this character is secondary and tertiary to the story line. While socio-economic diversity is found in Blackstone, many characters are poor. The wealthiest characters tend to be corrupt and their legitimate earnings arise from government work for the band.

Overall, these portrayals of older adults in current and popular television shows reveal that the depiction of older adults is becoming more nuanced, multidimensional and less stereotypical. Yet many of these depictions are still limited in their diversity. Because portrayals of characters in popular TV shows influence people's perceptions about themselves, their social groups and where they fit into society, it would be helpful if scriptwriters would not only maintain these non-traditional depictions of older people, but also bolster the diversity of the characters.

References

Altheide, D.L. (1987). Reflections: Ethnographic content analysis. *Qualitative Sociology* 10(1), 65–77.

Andriot, A. and Owens, T. (2012). Identity. *Oxford Bibliographies*. Retrieved from www.oxfordbibliographies.com/view/document/obo-9780199756384/obo-9780199756384-0025.xml.

Bazzini, D.G., McIntosh, W.D., Smith, S.M., Cook, S. and Harris, C. (1997). The aging women in popular film: Underrepresented, unattractive, unfriendly, and unintelligent. *Sex Roles* 36(7/8), 531–543.

Bell, J.S. (2004). *Write Great Fiction: Plot & structure*. Cincinnati, OH: Writer's Digest Books.

BBC News. (2013, March 18). TV viewing figures increase in UK. *BBC News*. Retrieved from www.bbc.com/news/entertainment-arts-21828961.

Branaman, A. (1997). Goffman's social theory. In C. Lemert and A. Branaman (eds). *The Goffman Reader*. Hoboken, NJ: Wiley-Blackwell.

Bureau of Labor Statistics. (2015). *American Time Use Survey*. Retrieved from www.bls.gov/tus.

Cardinal, G. (Writer) and Scott, R.E. (Director). (2011). *Future? What future?* [Television series. Season 1, Episode 1]. In R.E. Scott (Producer and Director). *Blackstone*. Canada: Prairie Dog Film & Television.

Esping-Andersen, G. (1990). *The Three Worlds of Welfare Capitalism*. Princeton, NJ: Princeton University Press.

Esping-Andersen, G. (1999). *Social Foundations of Post Industrial Economies*. New York: Oxford University Press.

Fellowes, J., Neame, G., Eaton, R. (Executive Producers). (2011). *Downton Abbey*. England: ITV Studios, Carnival Films.

Fellowes, J. (Writer) and Bolt, B. (Director). (2010). *Episode 2* [Television series. Season 1, Episode 2]. In J. Fellowes, G. Neame and R. Eaton (Executive Producers). *Downton Abbey*. England: ITV Studios, Carnival Films.

Fellowes, J. (Writer) and Percival, B. (Director). (2010). *Episode 1* [Television series. Season 1, Episode 1]. In J. Fellowes, G. Neame, R. Eaton (Executive Producers). (2011). *Downton Abbey*. England: ITV Studios, Carnival Films.

Goffman, E. (1963). *Stigma*. New York: Simon & Schuster.

Gran, B. (2008). Public of private management: A comparative analysis of social policies in Europe. *Sociological Compass 2(9)*, 1–29.

Howard, R., Grazer, B., Katims, J., Trilling, L., Watson, S., Nevins, D. (Executive Producers), Massin, D.K., Ward, P. and Goldberg, J. (Producers). (2013). *Parenthood*. Universal City, CA: Universal Media Studios, Universal Television, Imagine Television, Open 4 Business Productions.

Hudgins, D. (Writer) and Trilling, L. (Director). (2013). *All aboard who's coming aboard* [Television series. Season 5, Episode 2]. In R. Howard, B. Grazer, J. Katims, L. Trilling, S. Watson and D. Nevins (Executive Producers). *Parenthood*. Universal City, CA: Universal Media Studios, Universal Television, Imagine Television, Open 4 Business Productions.

Jenkins, R. (2014). *Self Identity*. London: Routledge.

Kauffman, M., Morris, H.J., Fonda, J., Tomlin, L., Weinstein, P., Goldberg, D., Ellison, D. and Ross, M. (Executive Producers). (2015a). *Grace and Frankie*. Santa Monica, CA: Skydance Television, Okay Goodnight.

Kauffman, M. and Morris, H.J. (Writers) and Taylor, T. (Director). (2015b). *The end* [Television series. Season 1, Episode 1]. In M. Kauffman, H.J. Morris, J. Fonda, L. Tomlin, P. Weinstein, D. Goldberg, D. Ellison and M. Ross (Executive Producers). *Grace and Frankie*. Santa Monica, CA: Skydance Television, Okay Goodnight.

Lutz, A. (2012, June 14). These corporations control 90% of the media in America. *Business Insider*. Retrieved from www.businessinsider.com/these-6-corporations-control-90-of-the-media-in-america-2012-6.

Marx, K. (1932). The German ideology. In J. Rivkin and M. Ryan (eds), *Literary Theory: An anthology* (pp. 653–658). Malden, MA: Blackwell Publishing.

Mead, G.H. (1934). *Mind, Self and Society*. In C.W. Morris (ed.). Chicago, IL: University of Chicago.

Mills, C.W. (1956). *The Power Elite*. Oxford: Oxford University Press.

Milner, C., Van Norman, K. and Milner, J. (2011). The media's portrayal of ageing. In: J.R. Beard, S. Biggs and D.E. Bloom (eds). *Global Population Ageing: Peril or promise*. Geneva: World Economic Forum.

Organisation for Economic Co-operation and Development (OECD). (2015). *Demography*. Retrieved from https://data.oecd.org/pop/elderly-population.htm.

Shindler, N. (Executive Producer). (2012). *Last Tango in Halifax*. England: Red Production Company.

Scott, R.E. (Producer and Director). (2011). *Blackstone*. Canada: Prairie Dog Film & Television.

Sneed, J.R. and Whitbourne, S.K. (2005). Models of the aging self. *Journal of Social Issues* 61(2): 375–388.

Television Bureau of Canada. (2015). *TV basics 2014–2015*. Retrieved from www. tvb.ca.

Vernon, J.A., Williams Jr., J.A., Phillips, T. and Wilson, J. (1990). Media stereotyping: A comparison of the way elderly women and men are portrayed on prime time television. *Journal of Women and Aging* 2(4), 55–68.

Vickers, K. (2007). Aging and the media: Yesterday, today, and tomorrow. *California Journal of Health Promotion* 5(3), 100–105.

Wainwright, S. (Writer) and Lyn, E. (Director). (2012a). *Episode 1* [Television series. Season 1, Episode 1]. In N. Shindler (Executive Producer). *Last Tango in Halifax*. England: Red Production Company.

Wainwright, S. (Writer) and Lyn, E. (Director). (2012b). *Episode 2* [Television series. Season 1, Episode 2]. In N. Shindler (Executive Producer). *Last Tango in Halifax*. England: Red Production Company.

Watson, S. (Writer) and Norris, P. (Director). (2013). *Nipple Confusion* [Television series. Season 5, Episode 3]. In R. Howard, B. Grazer, J. Katims, L. Trilling, S. Watson and D. Nevins (Executive Producers). *Parenthood*. Universal City, CA: Universal Media Studios, Universal Television, Imagine Television, Open 4 Business Productions.

3 Health-related technology use by older adults in rural and small town communities

Beth Perry, Margaret Edwards, Carol Anderson, Maiga Chang, Dr Kinshuk and Pamela Hawranik

This chapter explores how older adults living in rural and small town communities use technology for health-related purposes to remain healthy and live independently. Specifically, we explored if, and how, this population uses technology for health-related education, social support, health reminders (e.g. medication reminders), health alerts (e.g. texts to family if the person has fallen) and health parameter monitoring (e.g. blood pressure, pulse rate or breathing rate). The study is foundational to addressing questions related to effective use of technology for improving health self-care self-efficacy and maintenance of ability to independently perform activities of daily living in older adults. Data gathered include ways older adults use technology (mobile and home-based) for health-related purposes, access they have to health-related technology and ways older adults consider health-related technology helpful in assisting them to remain independent and community-dwelling.

A review of background literature, description of the research methods used, study findings and a discussion including recommendations for enhancing the use of health-related technology by older adults is included. The chapter concludes with recommendations for further research.

Background literature review

The number of older adults worldwide is growing due to factors such as an aging population, longer life expectancy and longer prognosis associated with chronic diseases (Kinsella et al., 2013). Additionally, restructuring healthcare in some countries places increased emphasis on home-based care, keeping older adults living in their own homes for as long as possible. Older adults with advanced illness or chronic conditions are increasingly community-dwelling rather than moving to institutionalized care (Stall et al., 2013). Increased community-dwelling places less strain on the institutional health system and independence is also the desire of many older adults who prefer to remain "at home" (Rosenberg, 2012).

The World Health Organization (2011) defines older adults as "people 60 years and older." "Rural and small town" populations consist of people "living in towns and municipalities outside the commuting zone of larger urban centres [which are] centres with populations of 10,000 or more" (Statistics Canada, 2001). In some rural and small town areas, there are insufficient numbers of institutional care facilities for older adults, fewer healthcare educational and support resources (Tryssenaar and Tremblay, 2002) and healthcare workers are more scarce (Park et al., 2009).

Older adults who reside in rural communities are especially vulnerable to negative health outcomes (Public Health Agency of Canada, 2010). This situation arises not only from their status as older adults but also through the potential compounding effects of rural residency. Innes et al. (2011) emphasize the need for more research regarding the impact of rurality on education and support requirements of rural residents. Health-related technology potentially brings effective and cost-effective solutions to help maintain health, well-being and independence in this vulnerable population.

Inefficiencies, increased demand and rising healthcare costs have severely crippled the healthcare system in many countries (Ghose, 2012). Jurisdictions are trying to reduce inefficiencies and meet demand by seeking better methods to deliver essential patient care services (Heckerman, 2009). Using health-related technology may help increase self-care self-efficacy, thus reducing the burden on the healthcare system. For example, non-invasive medical examination equipment can be used by individuals doing self-medical parameter monitoring (Tseng et al., 2007). The collected data can be transmitted to a central system via the Internet that returns the result and related information to the user (Chang et al., 2012). Many new, non-invasive mobile examination tools have been developed. For example, blood pressure, electrocardiogram, breath frequency and body temperature can be done by mobile devices (Koch, 2005). Blood glucose and international normalized ratios (INRs) can be home-monitored and results transmitted to physicians electronically (through the Virtual medical gend) for cost saving (Collen, 2000). Individuals are becoming more comfortable using technology for health-related purposes. For example, Seto et al. (2010) found heart failure patients were very comfortable using mobile phone-based remote monitoring.

Terry (2010) found that the quality and cost of mobile applications varies widely but concluded that smartphone applications have the potential to benefit the health and well-being of older adults. Contrary to stereotypical belief, recent research concludes that older adults are active users of the Internet and consumers of online information, with many expressing comfort with Internet-based technology (Mori and Harada, 2010). Gao and Koronios (2010) studied smartphone applications developed specifically for older adults to improve their life quality and concluded there was great potential but that more research was needed. Specifically, research focused on the use of technology by older adults to address educational, social support and health monitoring needs (Free et al., 2013).

Enhanced self-efficacy, adequate social support, the ability to call for help and receive expedient interventions when needed and consistent health parameter monitoring are linked to positive outcomes for populations (Spinsante et al., 2012). Low self-efficacy results in older adults lacking motivation to take actions toward maintaining their independence and levels of health. Likewise, perceived social support has also been linked to positive health outcomes. For example, Clark (2007) showed a positive correlation between social support in older adults and self-rated physical and mental health, and others found the same outcome for quality of life (Sherman et al., 2006). Essentially, adequate self-efficacy and perceived social support are linked to an improved sense of well-being and the potential for independence.

In sum, enhanced self-efficacy, perceived social support, health reminders and health parameter monitoring may have positive outcomes for the health and independence of older adults. These outcomes could lessen the strain on healthcare institutions and reduce related costs (Soderstrom et al., 2001). Institutionalized care may not be ideal for older people and many simply prefer to stay in their communities (Soderstrom et al., 2001). Using technology to educate, support, remind and monitor may help maintain the well-being of older adults, save healthcare resources and enhance quality of life for older adults.

Approach

This descriptive qualitative study elicited information from older adults living in rural and small town Alberta. A purposive convenience sample of older adults residing in three communities was recruited. From a list of older adult social clubs in Alberta, those groups from communities that met the definition of "rural or small town" (i.e., greater than 100km for a major urban centre) were selected for contact. The research assistant (RA) emailed the contact person from each qualifying social club explaining the study and asking if their group would be willing to participate in a focus group. From the 15 groups contacted, three agreed to participate. A total of 34 people participated in the focus groups with group sizes of 17, seven and ten people. Inclusion criteria included the ability to speak English, aged 60 years or older and consent to participate. Research ethics approval was obtained from the appropriate Research Ethics Review Board prior to commencing data collection.

A focus group was held in each participating community led by the RA who is a registered nurse with experience in data collection, care of older adults and administration in long-term care. Focus group sessions, held at a mutually agreeable time and place, lasted between one and two hours each and were audio-recorded and transcribed by the RA. Detailed notes were taken by the RA to supplement audio recordings. Each group began with a period of socialization where participants and the RA got acquainted over refreshments provided by the RA. Focus group sessions began by the RA obtaining consent from participants and ensuring that all participants met the inclusion criteria.

During the focus groups, questions regarding current availability, uses, functionality and fluency with health-related technology were asked. Further questions focused on perceived effects of health-related technology on health-related self-care self-efficacy, social support, health reminders and health parameter monitoring. Barriers to using technology for health-related purposes were discussed. The RA noted that participants were pleased to be selected for the study and noted that their opinions were rarely sought due to their geographic location.

Data were analyzed for themes using qualitative content analysis. The aim of qualitative content analysis is to condense data and produce a broad description of the phenomenon with categories describing the phenomenon (Elo and Kyngas, 2008). Content analysis began by the researchers' immersion in the data, followed by open coding where notes and headings were written on the transcripts. Categories were created bringing headings that were similar together. Then general categories or themes were determined from these headings. The themes are reported in this chapter. Data were coded and themes created by merging similar codes inductively (Elo and Kyngas, 2008).

Findings

Six themes emerged from the data, including types of technology used, primary uses of technology for health-related purposes, enthusiasm regarding use of technology for health-related purposes, desire for easy-to-learn technology and need for older, adult-friendly technology, frustration with access issues, and increased ability to choose to dwell in rural and small town communities. Each theme is discussed in the following sections using examples from transcript excerpts.

Theme one: types of technology used

The majority of participants owned mobile phones ranging from flip phones to smart phones to hands-free vehicle phones. Commonly, participants also owned computers (either laptop or desktop) and some owned tablets, although tablets were less common than other devices. Devices of all types were frequently shared between spouses. One person only carried her mobile phone in the winter for emergencies. Owning emergency call devices and health-monitoring technology (such as blood pressure monitors) was not common, but these devices were a technology priority for participants who had existing health issues. Opportunities for videoconferencing such as tele-health and videoconferencing workshops where experts from urban centres were available to consult on health or other issues were common in one community.

Theme two: primary uses of technology for health-related purposes

Older adult participants used mobile phones, tablets, laptops and personal computers for several health-related purposes, including staying in touch with family and friends, researching health information and for self-care health advice. There was limited use of technology for medication reminders, heath parameter monitoring and recording, or health alerts. Each use is explored in more detail.

Staying in touch: the children and grandchildren factor

Devices of all types were primarily used for staying in touch with family and friends. This social purpose was the most frequent use of technology and the most common driver to purchase and learn to use technology. Literature links maintenance of strong social connections with good health, especially social-emotional well-being. For example, Cohen and Wills' (1985) stress and coping social support theory emphasizes the stress buffering effects of social support and correlates reduced stress with increased health.

One group of participants commented that 90 percent of their technology use is for "communication and sharing photographs." Facebook, email, texting, Skype and telephoning were methods used to make contact, share photos, arrange meeting times and places, share concerns, ask questions and offer and receive advice and support. Facebook was the least popular strategy; texting and Skype were most commonly used. Participants frequently relied on technology to stay in touch when traveling or when living apart from family and friends. They noted that using texting to stay in touch was "much cheaper than using the phone." Some also used two technologies synergistically (e.g., texting grandchildren before calling them on the phone to determine if it was a good time to call). Other participants noted they receive but do not send text messages, making texting one-way communication for them. One person had a Twitter account and no one mentioned blogging. One adult learning society affiliated with a participant community reported that the most frequent request they receive is for courses on email and social media as well as for help with downloading and uploading photographs.

Grandchildren, children and other younger friends played several important roles in the successful use of technology by participants. Specifically, they motivated older adults to use technology for social communication and often became teachers and tech support for older adults who used technology. Several participants noted "the kids do it" when talking about purchasing, setting up, troubleshooting and upgrading their technology. One participant commented that she had just bought a tablet but did not know how to use it so she invited a "young fellow to dinner and told him I'd feed him dinner if he would come and give me a lesson on how to use it." Another noted, "kids are much more adept at using technology ... they grew up with it, we didn't."

Family and friends were also motivation for using technology for communication, connection and socialization. Participants commented that they wanted to stay in touch with children and grandchildren so felt it was effective to use their language/medium of communication. One woman said she learned to text because the kids do. Several noted that their children no longer have landline telephones, and, if they do have landlines, they do not answer the phone. Consequently, participants said they had to learn to text to be in touch with them. As one commented, "I had to learn to text to stay in touch with my daughter because you can never get a hold of her any other way." Another said of her adult children, "they don't actually talk on the phone ... they never answer a regular phone."

Some study participants reported wanting to see photos of grandchildren who lived far away and technology provided them a route to see their family members. For example, Skype was a way of watching a grandchild grow up without being physically present. One participant commented she learned to Skype to "see the kids." Another taught his grandson to speak German using Skype, facilitating a familial connection and "keeping his culture going." In another instance, the participant's granddaughter taught the grandmother to use her Blackberry through Skype. In sum, technology use was motivated and facilitated by family and friends and the resulting social connections older adult participants found to be health promoting.

Researching health information and self-care health advice

The second common use for devices was researching health information including drug information, diagnosis, symptoms and self-care health advice. Almost all participants used Google as their search engine. Even the people who admitted they were uneasy regarding using technology admitted they "Google."

Participants commented they used the Internet to supplement health information from healthcare practitioners. For example, following a doctor's visit, participants said they look up their condition or medications on the Internet to help them with unanswered questions and to enhance understanding. As one commented, "the doctor gives you a report with all these words on it and you don't have a clue what they mean and he doesn't have time to explain it ... I go to sites like Mayo Clinic or Rochester or Alberta Health Services to find out what he said." Participants said they preferred medical websites that provide health information "straight up and in plain language."

As older adults become increasingly well-educated consumers, taking ownership of their healthcare, they will want additional health information which the Internet and technology can provide. Participants reported that if a health issue was bothering them, they often looked up the symptoms on the Internet before seeking medical advice. Further, they "Googled" side effects of medications to avoid calling the pharmacist. They reported a desire to look after their own health to remain in control of health matters and to achieve independent living for as long as possible.

A common concern among participants was how to determine if the health information they obtained on the Internet was credible and valid. They noted they have developed strategies for checking the quality of what they read on the Internet. One said, "I always look it up twice and see if I get the same meaning two times." Another participant agreed saying, "I find more than one site for sure," and then she described how she compares sites to ensure they are in agreement. If the content on sites was consistent, older adults in the study believed the information. However, they remained cautious regarding their ability to assess the quality of Internet sites.

Some participants commented that they often found different sites "say something different about the same health question" and they are left wondering "who to believe" and "how do you know which one is right." All participants expressed a sense of carefulness agreeing that "you can't believe everything you read on the Internet." Focus group participants noted that education regarding how to evaluate the quality of a health website would be of great interest to them.

Participants reported that their doctors were not always encouraging of their use of the Internet to look up health information. One disclosed her doctor said, "don't go on the computer!" when cautioning her about seeking outside information about her symptoms. Almost all participants said they proceed to use the Internet to seek health advice and check symptoms even when their healthcare professionals discourage it, although they are reluctant to admit this to their care providers.

Using technology to overcome limitations and remain independent

Some participants explained they used technology to overcome health-related limitations, such as reduced physical mobility or no longer being able to drive. For example, one 80 year old uses online banking. Her mobility was compromised due to physical changes. Online shopping was not common among participants, but some said it was within their range of possibilities for the future to obtain groceries and other daily needs. In these ways, technology was helping them remain independent and not relying on others for transportation. Participants reported psychological health benefits to independence.

More specific to health monitoring, a limited number of participants reported using home blood pressure (BP) monitors which allowed them to frequently screen these values without needing access to medical facilities. If abnormal values were detected at home they could seek medical help expediently, possibly avoiding morbidity. As one participant said of mobile monitoring devices, "they allow me to monitor myself … to look after myself." When the RA introduced the possibility of monitoring INRs at home using systems such as CoaguChek (CoaguChek, n.d.), participants who were taking anticoagulants were very interested in exploring the possibility of purchasing this technology. They commented that the main advantage of home monitoring was "staying healthy" so they could remain independent.

Theme three: enthusiasm regarding using technology for health-related purposes

Participants were clear that they want to continue to use technology and be involved in what is current in this field. They were positive about both current and potential benefits of technology for them. One primary benefit they perceived was increased opportunity to continue to live in their rural or small town community rather than moving to urban centres where health services are readily available. Participants seemed especially keen to learn more about using technology that would help them achieve the goal of remaining independent and community-dwelling. This strong desire seemed to fuel their enthusiasm for technology.

When the RA provided examples of various health technologies such as tele-health, smart phone medication reminders, mobile devices for monitoring vital signs and automatic transmission of abnormal findings to their healthcare team, participants commented that they were not very familiar with most of these uses of technology. However, they almost universally expressed interest in learning about these uses of technology and said they would use them if they were available. Participants brainstormed ideas during the focus groups regarding how they could find out more about available health-related technology and stressed they understood the need to become informed consumers. Some participants commented they planned to talk with their doctors about what health technology might be applicable to them, and others considered the possibility of planning a trade show in their community where vendors would showcase health technology products.

While participants were excited about meaningful uses of health-related technology, they expressed little patience for technology they did not deem useful. For example, when discussing Facebook one person said, "I'm not fond of it. Someone compared it to the old party line … they put pictures on there and talk about what they are going to have for supper … who cares?" There was general agreement among focus group attendees that sharing personal details with "strangers" was not their priority use of technology and that it did not contribute to their health.

While enthusiastic about using technology, participants agreed that it was often lack of confidence that prevented them from learning to use it. One woman said, "I don't have the confidence since my stroke … I feel like I am not going to learn." Another supposed, "confidence is huge for any of us ... my daughter said, 'just push buttons Mom, you can't hurt it'" but another participant quickly suggested that "was not good advice." The older adult participants wanted to continue to learn to use technology to its full potential, and saw health benefits, but some needed support and encouragement to do so.

Participants reported they provide support to one another related to technology use. They were impressed by their peers who were competent with technology and expressed a desire to increase their own technology competence. One participant noted that a peer had his smart phone set with reminders for garbage pick-up dates, etc. As the participant said of this man, "he's got everything on his phone ... he's got it beeping all the time." While the participants were impressed with peers who were using technology, and they admitted their own lack of skill in this area, they generally were not afraid to learn more and to start using technology for health-related purposes.

Interestingly, participants used humour to cover current lack of skill and knowledge regarding use of technology. Alongside their growing confidence in technology use, participants readily admitted their relative incompetence with some applications. During the focus groups they kibitzed among themselves and with the RA regarding their limitations with using their devices. For example, one said with excitement on being shown a Blackberry tablet by another person at the focus group, "that's a Blackberry too? Well for heaven's sake. I thought they were little things. That must be one of the newer ones then." The comment caused laughter in the group including the person who made the comment. Another participant noticed during the focus group that he had a message on his smart phone and announced with a smile, "oh, I have a message ... you'd better stop the meeting so I can check it." The recipient then observed that the message had been sent many months earlier. Again the group laughed together at this admission. While they laughed at themselves regarding their technology knowledge deficit, they simultaneously expressed a desire to become competent.

Theme four: desire for easy to learn and need for older adult-friendly technology

Participants noted that they want technology that is simple to learn and to use. One woman expressed that her current smart phone was too complicated for her to ever learn to use. Specifically, she thought there were too many steps to making a call and too many uses in one device. Participants suggested that often the fonts are too small, making reading messages challenging. Others noted that the keys were too close together making texting awkward.

Participants viewed using technology as a good use of their time. As they said, "it occupies time and that's good ... we are not just sitting in front of a TV ... we are learning stuff when we are on the Internet. It is more interactive. We are not just being force fed." In other words, the older adults valued the opportunity to choose topics, sources and format (written or video). They enjoyed asking questions and sharing what they were learning, making the online experience interactive.

Theme five: frustration with access issues

Some participants commented that living in rural areas and small towns meant that they had lack of choice of provider, inconsistency with reliability of access and limited Internet access, which they found frustrating. For example, only dial-up was available from one major provider in one small town setting in the study. Another provider in the same town did offer satellite and wireless options but access tended to be sporadic. Participants in one focus group reported that their Internet went "down" approximately three times per week and that they often got a "no signal" message. One participant said, "our calls keep getting dropped and we don't have good access." They reported one supplier recommended they not move to smart phones because they would not function reliably in their community. Participants reported that they did have reliable Internet in their local library and hospital but not at their homes. Although frustrated with limited Internet access and cell coverage, they were willing to accept this limitation to live their preferred rural and small town lifestyle. However, they noted that their adult children regarded the access issue as one reason they should consider moving to an urban centre.

Not all rural and small town communities have the same experience with Internet access and reliability. One of the communities in the study was also home to a post-secondary institution and an affiliated continuing education facility for adults, offering courses related to using technology and also offering videoconference workshops. This same community was home to eight churches that used technology. Participants from this community recognized that they were influenced by their connections with these community institutions and that, as a result, they were exposed to uses of technology and were "early adopters" of technology for their own purposes. Participants expressed that they experienced "less fear" in using technology as it was "more common" in their community. This example shows there is inconsistency with technology access among rural and small town communities.

Participants also commented that access was limited by a lack of financial resources for some older adults. As one said of technology, "cost can be prohibitive for those on fixed incomes." Additionally, participants pointed out that the cost of satellite Internet (which provided them with better delivery and more reliable service) was much more than other available Internet options (approximately $20.00/month more). Older adults reported making use of places in their towns where there was open access Internet because having it in their homes was "too big a chunk out of their income." Another cost issue noted by participants was the cost of staying current, as well as the pressure to "keep up with the Joneses and have the latest technology," which resulted in an access issue for some. Further, although health monitoring devices such as CoaguChek were seen as helpful by participants, they noted that if the cost of such devices was not covered by health insurance, it could be too expensive for them.

Theme six: technology enhances ability to choose to dwell in home communities

Participants expressed a desire to use technology to further their individual determination, choice over where they live and how they live their lives. They believed that technology could help them retain their rural and small town life, while giving them access to urban expertise and healthcare. Technology in their estimation could reduce the potential disparity between quality of healthcare in urban and other settings.

A difference in access and reliability of technology in rural and small town communities was a concern for the participants. They expressed a willingness to sacrifice access to technology for the rural and small town lifestyle but they wanted to become more self-sufficient in terms of technology. Tele-health was available to some to provide access to urban physicians without older adults having to leave their communities. Some participants had experienced tele-health (e.g., sending EKG strips from a pacemaker for interpretation in real-time during a cardiac assessment). One community had a local adult learning society that offered videoconferencing workshops, their local library had audio and e-books and their physicians used tele-health to connect with consultants from the city. In other communities, such use of technology was more limited. In sum, community-dwelling was their goal and technology was seen as a tool to help achieve this goal.

Discussion

The themes described above give rise to strategies and recommendations for enhancing the use of health-related technology by older adults living in rural and small town settings. These strategies and recommendations are as follows.

Develop and make available appropriate older, adult-friendly devices

While participants were keen to use technology, they also expressed a desire for simple-to-use devices. One group suggested devices with three or four functions instead of a menu of choices. Another called for devices with bigger keys commenting, "my fingers are just a little large sometimes." One participant owned a store that sells technological devices and he observed that he gets frequent requests from older adult customers who want "a basic phone for basic communication." He concluded, "there is a need for simpli-fication" of devices. Participants expressed enthusiasm for current devices that allow font size adjustment. Participants also noted that there is lack of education for older adults regarding what is available in terms of technol-ogy that meets their specific needs. Therefore, a market opportunity exists for developers to create more technological devices with fewer features and larger interfaces. Regular education about procurement and use of devices with special emphasis on devices that are available that are older adult friendly in design and function is suggested.

Beyond more streamlined devices in terms of functions and age appropri-ate fonts, etc., education related to what technology is available to help with issues encountered by some older adults is required. While participants were very interested in using technology, they noted they were not aware of some technologies available. For example, many did not know about technology that would allow them to monitor INR values at home. Regularly scheduled information sessions about new technological products and devices that might help them maintain their health and remain community-dwelling was suggested by participants.

Need for ongoing older adult education regarding credible health information and how to use this information effectively

One common concern expressed by study participants was assessing the credibility and validity of online health information. Participants noted they were interested in learning information assessment strategies. This finding alerts us to the need for older, adult-friendly education regarding assess-ment of health information found on the Internet. Ongoing education on this topic, using pedagogy appropriate for this age group, is recommended. Educational sessions should be offered at times and places convenient for older adult learners.

Further, study participants wanted to learn how to use the "good" information they find on the Internet to augment their interactions with healthcare providers. More specifically, they wanted to be informed con-sumers of healthcare information, working collaboratively with physicians, nurses, pharmacists and other healthcare providers to help themselves maintain optimum health. Participants believed that being well-informed by credible online health information prepared them to ask important ques-tions and make informed health choices in discussion with health caregivers. Again, effective education, including collaboration strategies, could help older adults meet this goal.

Participants said they wanted healthcare professionals to help guide them in seeking credible health information online and they wanted these profes-sionals to be receptive to discussing their findings. In sum, older adults in the study wanted their professional partners to be supportive and receptive to their uses of health-related technology.

Reduce cost or subsidy of Internet and data plans for older adults

In terms of access to online information and purchasing of devices and data plans, some older adults noted the financial cost was limiting. If access to health information and monitoring can reduce the need for institutionalization of older adults and help them maintain optional health-negating visits to healthcare providers and facilities, then it could be cost effective to the healthcare system to subsidize device purchase and Internet access fees. For example, if enhanced knowledge and monitoring and effective health reminders decrease morbidity in older adults, they will have fewer emergency room visits, may require less medication and might remain community-dwelling longer. These outcomes would all have a positive impact on healthcare costs as well as potentially on the well-being of the older adults.

Plan communities for older adults to include Internet access

Since older adults want to be technologically current and connected, communities where older adults reside should have Internet access addressed in community design and construction. For example, each older adult housing unit should have wireless Internet access. Public spaces in older adult communities should have community computers for use by residents. Libraries, coffee shops and other community spaces should encourage older adults to stay connected by providing free Internet access and perhaps computer hardware and educational sessions on use of technology as well.

More research related to effective pedagogy for teaching technology to older adults

As increasing numbers of older adults seek to learn to use technology, educational strategies focused on effective teaching for this group will need to be designed. Participants in this study noted that for them, 1:1 learning was the most effective. They preferred to learn about one use of each device per instruction session and then to have a chance to practice that skill before moving to a different use of technology. Further, participants commented that timing of instruction was important. That is, learning something that they had a current need to use was more effective than learning a skill they would not use until sometime in the future. Educators specialized in teaching older adults might be the most skilled at coaching this group as they would be sensitive to assessing educational needs, learning styles and readiness to learn, as well as to creating educational programing that would facilitate learning. Further research is needed focused on creating educational programs for supporting older adults who want to use technology so that they can do so confidently.

Conclusion

Older adults desire to be informed health consumers remaining in control of their health and living independently in their chosen locations. Technology may play a role in helping them secure reliable health information, stay connected to significant supports and remain independent. Indeed, the roles for technology in health maintenance of older adults will likely continue to expand. The study participants already saw the value of technology for good health saying, "we are not afraid of technology for health. There are immediate benefits."

The major outcome of this study is knowledge related to uses of health-related technology to enhance the health, well-being and independence of older adults living in rural and small town communities. Focus group participants provided examples of how they use technology to stay connected with others, research health information and self-care advice, and overcome barriers to living independently in locations of their choice. Participants expressed concerns regarding access issues. Older adults in this study articulated interest in using technology for health-related outcomes and expressed a desire to become increasingly technologically savvy. Strategies for enhancing the use of health-related technologies with this population are detailed.

Further research related to health-related technology use by older adults in rural and small town communities is needed to expand the study findings. This descriptive exploratory study provides foci for further investigation. Investigations related to effective pedagogy for older adults and studies evaluating form and function of technological devices and programs that enhance usability from the older adult perspective could inform technology development. Research-based assessment of the health benefits of using health-related technology in this population could help justify financial investment in devices, education and support, and related infrastructure.

The research reported in this chapter adds to existing knowledge in gerontology in several ways. First, it details ways that older adults living in rural and small town situations use health-related technology to assist them in remaining healthy, independent and community-dwelling. It notes the barriers that these older adults face in using health-related technologies and it provides strategies and recommendations for enhancing the use of health-related technology by older adults living in rural and small town situations. With respect to practice and the nursing care of older people, our findings suggest that many older adults want to use technology for health-related purposes and many need the encouragement and support of nurses to do so. Nurses and other care providers may contribute to helping inform older adults who use technology and can assist them in finding health information regarding how to assess the quality of Internet references and resources. Nurses should learn to collaborate with older adults who want to use technology to become informed healthcare consumers.

This study also provides a foundation for further research and policy, addressing questions related to effective use of technology for improving health self-care self-efficacy and maintaining the ability of older adults to live independently in rural and small town communities. Findings support need for further development of health-related technologies, specifically for older adults. Research focused on the use of technology by older adults could help to address the educational, social support and health monitoring needs of this vulnerable population.

References

Chang, M., Heh, J.S. and Lin, H.N. (2012). Tele-physical examination and tele-care systems for elderly people. *Journal of Community Informatics*, 8(1). Retrieved from http://ci-journal.net/index.php/ciej/article/view/762/900.

Clark, K. (2007). *The Influence of Social Support on Health for Chronically-Ill Urban and Rural Seniors from Three Canadian Provinces* (unpublished Master's thesis). University of Western Ontario, Canada.

CoaguChek (n.d.). *CoaguChek System Website*. Retrieved from www.coaguchek. com.

Cohen, S. and Wills, T.A. (1985). Stress, social support, and the buffering hypothesis. *Psychological Bulletin*, *98*, 310–357.

Collen, M.F. (2000). Historical evolution of preventive medical informatics in the USA. *Methods of Information in Medicine*, *39*(3), 204–207.

Elo, S. and Kyngas, H. (2008). The qualitative content analysis process. *Journal of Advanced Nursing*, *62*(1), 107–115.

Free, C., Phillips, G., Watson, L., Galli, L., Felix, L., Edwards, P., Patel, V. and Haines, A. (2013). The effectiveness of mobile-health technologies to improve health care service delivery processes: A systematic review and meta-analysis. *PLOS Medicine*, *10*(1), 1–26.

Gao, J. and Koronios, A. (2010). *Mobile Application Development for Senior Citizens*. Pacific Asia Conference on Information Systems (PACIS) 2010 Proceedings. Paper 65. Taipei, Taiwan, July 9–12.

Ghose, T. (2012). Canada needs (and can afford) complete national health care. *CCPA Monitor*, *19*(7), 18–20.

Heckerman, D. (2009). Healthcare delivery in developing countries: Challenges and potential solutions. In T. Hey, S. Tansley and K. Tolle (eds). *The Fourth Paradigm*. Redmond, WA: Microsoft Research.

Innes, A., Morgan, D. and Kosteniuk, J. (2011). Dementia care in rural and remote settings: A systematic review of informal/family caregiving. *Maturitas*, *69*(2), 34–46.

Kinsella, K., Beard, J. and Suzman, R. (2013). Can populations age better, not just live longer? *Generations*, *37*(1), 19–26.

Koch, S. (2005). Home telehealth: Current state and future trends. *International Journal of Medical Informatics*, *75*(8), 565–576.

Mori, K. and Harada, E. (2010). Is learning a family matter? Experimental study of the influence of social environment on learning by older adults in the use of mobile phones. *Japanese Psychological Research*, *52*(3), 244–255.

Park, E., Do, S., Shin, H. and Nam, H.S. (2009). *An Adaptive Streaming Technique for Interactive Medical Systems in Mobile Environment.* Proceedings of the 6th International Conference on Mobile Technology, Application & Systems, Nice, France, September 2–4.

Public Health Agency of Canada (2010). Retrieved from www.phac-aspc.gc.ca/cphorsphc-respcacsp/2010/fr-rc/cphorsphc-respcacsp-06-eng.php

Rosenberg, T. (2012). Acute hospital use, nursing home placement, and mortality in a frail community-dwelling cohort managed with primary integrated interdisciplinary elder care at home. *Journal of the American Geriatrics Society*, 60(7), 1340–1346.

Seto, E., Leonard, K.J., Masino, C., Cafazzo, J.A., Barnsley, J. and Ross, H.J. (2010). Attitudes of heart failure patients and health care providers towards mobile phone-based remote monitoring. *Journal of Medical Internet Research*, 12(4). Retrieved from www.jmir.org/2010/4/e55

Sherman, A.M., Shumaker, S.A., Rejeski, W.J., Morgan, T., Applegate, W.B. and Ettinger, W. (2006). Social support, social integration, and health-related quality of life over time: Results from the fitness and arthritis in seniors trial (FAST). *Psychology & Health*, 21(4), 463–480.

Soderstrom, L., Tousignant, P. and Kaufman, T. (2001). Acute? Care at home: The health and cost effects of substituting home care for inpatient acute care: A review of the evidence. *Journal of the American Geriatrics Society*, 49(8), 1123–1126.

Spinsante, S., Antonicelli, R., Mazzanti, I. amd Gambi, E. (2012). Technological approaches to remote monitoring of elderly people in cardiology: A usability perspective. *International Journal of Telemedicine & Applications*, 2012, 1–10.

Stall, N., Nowaczynski, M. and Sinha, S.K. (2013). Back to the future: Home-based primary care for older homebound Canadians: Part 2: Where we are going? *Canadian Family Physician*, 59, 243–245.

Statistics Canada. (2001). *Rural and Small Town Canada Analysis Bulletin*, 3(3). Catalogue no. 21-006-XIE. Retrieved from www.statcan.gc.ca/pub/21-006-x/21-006-x2001003-eng.pdf.

Terry, M. (2010). Medical apps for smartphones. *Telemedicine and e-Health*, 16(1), 17–22.

Tryssenaar, J. and Tremblay, M. (2002). Aging with a serious mental disability in rural Northern Ontario: Family members' experiences. *Psychiatric Rehabilitation Journal*, 25(2), 255–265.

Tseng, C.H., Lin, H.N., Cheng, S.Y., Heh, J.S. and Lo, W.M. (2007). *Clinical Alert Mechanism Based on X-Chart in Physical Signal Examination System.* Proceedings of the 14th International Congress of Oriental Medicine, (ICOM 2007), Taipei, Taiwan, December 2–4, No. 0081.

World Health Organization. (2011). *Definition of an Older or Elderly Person.* Retrieved from www.who.int/healthinfo/survey/ageingdefnolder/en/index.html.

4 Relationship between physical/ psychological predictors and self-rated health among older people in Hong Kong

Shelly Kin Shan Leung, Linda Chiu Wa Lam, Oi Ling Siu and Gillian Joseph

Studies have shown repeatedly that an individual's *subjective* evaluation of overall health is an important indicator of her/his *objective* health status (Pan and Ward, 2015). Self-rated health (SRH), or global SRH, is a form of self-evaluation in which research participants are asked to compare their current health status to a reference level, often using a Likert-type scale. This self-evaluation goes beyond simply reporting illness to elicit information about participants' deeper reflections on the subtle biological and physiological changes that affect a sense of well-being. This information can be used to both track changes in specific populations across time and to characterize differences between populations (Pan and Ward, 2015).

In recent years, the World Health Organization (WHO), along with health authorities in many countries, has advocated for a greater emphasis to be placed on the subjective dimension within research on population health (World Health Organization, 2015). To some extent, a positive response to this call to embrace the subjective dimension of health is already evident, such that it is no longer unusual to find self-rated health incorporated in epidemiological investigations. In large part, this "shift to the subjective" reflects a growing recognition that self-rated health can be a robust predictor of future disability and mortality (World Health Organization, 2015; see also Haring et al., 2011; Idler and Kasl, 1995). Indeed, nearly two decades ago, Idler and Benyamini (1997) reported findings from 27 studies across 12 countries that showed that global SRH is a good predictor of mortality, independent of other physical, behavioral or psychosocial risk factors. The practical importance of measuring SRH was further highlighted in a meta-analytic study reported by Desalvo et al. (2006) in which it was found that individuals who rated their health as "poor" had a two-fold higher risk of mortality than those who reported their health as "excellent," even after controlling for comorbidity and other risk factors.

Looking across what is now an extensive body of scholarship, it is possible to identify three commonly cited predictors of SRH: the presence or absence of (i) physical illness, (ii) functional disability and (iii) depressive symptoms (Hays et al., 1996; Idler and Kasl, 1995). Other factors that have been found repeatedly to be associated with poorer SRH include subjective cognitive impairment (Walker et al., 2004) and negative affect (Mulsant et al., 1997; Segerstrom, 2013). However, while important insights have been gained through studies aimed at identifying the contributing or predictive factors for SRH, the completeness of existing models has been called into question. For example, very few studies have examined the relative importance of mechanisms that underlie the predictive factors for SRH. In turn, while SRH is understood to underlie a number of conditions ranging from the physical to the psychological, the objective to the subjective and the clinical to the prodromal (Idler and Benyamini, 1997), the clear identification of linkages between them has been elusive. We address this deficiency in the study presented later in this chapter.

Numerous studies have shown that advanced age, poor functional ability, depressive symptoms, a high number of physical illnesses and a high level of subjective cognitive impairments are associated with poor SRH. Comorbidity is thus a phenomenon that researchers need to take into consideration when examining the predictive factors for SRH, particularly in populations of older adults, as the number of medical conditions tends to increase with age (Canadian Institute of Health Information, 2011). The untangling of threads of causality are further complicated by the fact that the effects of individual predictors on SRH can be either direct or indirect, or both. For example, the negative impact of increasing age on SRH has been found to be mediated by functional ability (Hirve et al., 2014). Similarly, changes in comorbidity have been found to be associated with poorer SRH, although this relationship is nonlinear and moderated by age and baseline comorbidity (Heller et al., 2009).

In addition to the lack of specificity with respect to the indirect-versus-direct impact of potential predictors on SRH, concerns have also been expressed with respect to the possible existence of conjoint relationships among predictors. Stenback (1964) coined the term *coenaesthesis* to describe a *whole-body feeling*—suggesting that all sensations considered together by an individual constitutes more than the sum of its parts. While coenaesthesis arguably represents an extreme form within overlapping and interwoven patterns of relationship, it does suggest that simple approaches to SRH, such as focusing on the additive effect of symptoms, may be insufficient as a means of accounting for variations in SRH within populations. Complexity needs to be embraced. By way of illustration, objective conditions, such as advanced age or physical illness, can directly influence SRH, while at the same time these conditions may limit the influence exerted by clinical conditions such as depression. Conversely, the presence of depressive symptoms may have an amplifying effect when objective health problems are also present (Segerstrom, 2013).

The study

Hong Kong is the most rapidly aging jurisdiction in Asia (Phillips et al., 2005) and this makes this Special Administrative Region (SAR) of China an attractive location for studies of aging. In this chapter, we seek to both contribute to local knowledge of aging and to advance general understanding of the subjective dimensions of health by developing and presenting a comprehensive model for describing the associations between SRH and a number of physical and psychological predictors among Hong Kong's aging population.

Two versions of SRH are operationalized in the study. The first draws on Social Identity Theory, originally developed by Tajfel and Turner in 1994 (Marques et al., 2015; Tajfel and Turner, 1979). Social identity theory postulates that people's identities are partly rooted in their memberships of social groups and categories and that this identity can have important consequences for self-esteem, well-being and health (e.g. Falomir-Pichastor et al., 2009; Haslam et al., 2009; Jones et al., 2011). Thus the first measure of SRH we use is based on participants comparing their current health to that of others (SRH compared to others). The second uses a measure of SRH based upon individuals' views of changes to their own health over time: "SRH compared to last year."

Similar studies to ours have been rare in China or in jurisdictions in which an ethnic Chinese population predominates. Moreover, we are not aware of any studies that have adopted a measure that asks participants to compare their subjective health to that of others. We regard the use of this measure as a major contribution to the scholarship on this topic.

Considering that approximately one-fifth of the world's population is Chinese, exploring SRH in a jurisdiction whose population is predominantly (94 percent) ethnic Chinese (Hong Kong Census and Statistics Department, 2011) holds promise for generalizing findings to a wider population. Self-reported health has sometimes been criticized for its lack of consideration of cultural factors that may explain differences in results across populations (Pan and Ward, 2015; World Health Organization, 2015). The demographic makeup of Hong Kong therefore serves as an ideal population from which assumptions can be drawn and reliably generalized to other Chinese populations. We see this as a second major contribution to scholarship on the subjective dimensions of health.

Finally, using data from a large study of clinical records collected by the Government of the Hong Kong SAR's Department of Health constitutes a further contribution to the study of this topic. The use of Health Department data has a twofold benefit. First, it will make the use of results more likely, in terms of both dealing with the practical challenges of assessing health in Hong Kong and in highlighting the potential contribution of particular supports and services that could assist in improving the health of its aging population. Second, the use of Health Department data allows our study to be replicated in other parts of the SAR.

Hypotheses

Prior to the collection and analysis of data on SRH, we drew from the literature four testable hypotheses that capture key questions about the determinants of SRH, and that also have relevance to discussions of health-care provision in Hong Kong. The specific rationale for each hypothesis is summarized below.

Hypothesis 1: older age will be associated with poorer SRH

In view of the success of SRH in predicting future disability and mortality, a growing number of studies have attempted to identify the predictors of SRH itself. First, some studies have suggested that SRH may worsen with increased age. For example, in a population-based study of 27,757 people aged 18–80 years, older people were found to have higher odds ratios of poor SRH (Lindström, 2009). In other words, age and SRH were negatively correlated. Similarly, a study of more than 37,000 employees in Taiwan found that older workers were more likely to report poor SRH, which was attributed in part to the presence of symptoms of multiple diseases (Cheng et al., 2013). Therefore, we hypothesize that in a cross-sectional analysis, SRH will be poorer for older age groups.

Hypothesis 2: the reporting of a higher degree of physical illness will be associated with poorer SRH

SRH is known to be associated with physical health status, with poor physical health being a significant contributor to poor SRH (Idler and Benyamini, 1997). It has also been shown that higher levels of chronic disease are predictive of poorer SRH (Segerstrom, 2013; Zavras et al., 2013). In turn, difficulties in physical and cognitive functioning have been shown longitudinally to predict declining health (Benyamini et al., 2011). In light of these studies, we hypothesize that in a cross-sectional analysis, SRH will be poorer among those reporting multiple illnesses.

Hypothesis 3: the reporting of more depressive symptoms will be associated with poorer SRH

Evidence suggests that depression is significantly associated with poorer SRH in all age groups (French et al., 2012), and that it is an independent risk factor for subsequent changes in SRH in older adults (Han, 2002). For instance, a longitudinal study of people with a functional disability revealed that a decrease in depressive symptoms was associated with decreased odds of a decline in SRH (Han and Jylha, 2006). Furthermore, physical and mental health conditions at baseline can predict future changes in SRH. Verropoulou (2012) reported that after a three-year interval, SRH was related to the number of baseline chronic illnesses and depressive symptoms. Similarly, in a group of 150 community-dwelling, married adults over the age of 60, differences in negative affect were found to predict poorer SRH (Segerstrom, 2013). Overall, we hypothesize that in a cross-sectional analysis, SRH will be poorer among those reporting a high number of depressive symptoms.

Hypothesis 4: more exercise will be associated with better SRH

SRH has also been found to be significantly related to physical activity (Kerr et al., 2012; Parkatti et al., 1998), echoing the fact that such activity has been shown to reduce the risk of numerous chronic diseases, including cardiovascular disease, obesity and diabetes (World Health Organization, 1990). Lee (2000) reported that good physical fitness could lower the risk of functional decline and mortality, while Tran et al. (2013) reported that moderate and vigorous physical activity has a similar positive association with SRH status. In a longitudinal study, a more active physical life was found to be associated with lower health decline, after controlling for socio-demographic variables (Benyamini et al., 2011), while low levels of physical activity were found to be significantly related to a decline in SRH (Verropoulou, 2012). Taking this evidence into account, we hypothesize that in a cross-sectional analysis, SRH will be better among those reporting greater amounts of exercise.

Approach

We conducted a large-scale, community-based retrospective cohort study using baseline clinical record data provided by the Government of the Hong Kong SAR Department of Health.

Elderly Health Centres (EHC) were established throughout Hong Kong by the Department of Health to cater specifically to elderly residents aged 65 or over. Like all the EHCs, the Nam Sham Clinic offers a range of services, including annual physical check-ups, health assessments and treatments.

Anonymized data were retrieved from the clinical record database for group analyses. To be included in the study, older adults were required to have used the services at the Nam Shan EHC since 2005 and to have had at least two follow-up assessments there between 2006 and 2011, with at least one of the follow-up assessments having occurred since 2008. Eligibility was restricted to community-dwelling ethnic Chinese aged 65 or over, with no known history of cerebrovascular accidents or dementia at the time of attending Nam Shan EHC in 2005. Participants residing in old-age homes or with a history of cerebrovascular accidents were excluded. Participants with significant cognitive impairment (SCI) were also excluded. SCI was defined by the presence of clinical dementia, or a sub-threshold score on the Cantonese version of the Mini-Mental State Examination (C-MMSE): ≤ 18

for illiterate participants, ≤20 for those with 1–2 years of education or ≤22 for those with more than two years of education. After screening, information on 2,046 participants was included in our study.

Personal information and measurements were drawn from the clinical records of the Nam Shan EHC for use in the study. These are summarized below.

Demographic characteristics—Information on gender, age, date of birth, type of housing, marital status and educational level was included.

SRH—As noted earlier, two measures of SRH were used in the study. Participants had first been asked to compare their current health with that of others (SRH compared to others) in a three-item Likert Scale as either: "better than others" (1), "similar to others" (2) or "worse than others" (3). Participants were then asked to compare their current health to their own health status in the previous year (SRH compared to oneself last year) as: "better than last year" (1), "similar to last year" (2) or "worse than last year" (3). In both measures, a higher score indicates a lower level of SRH.

Physical illnesses—Participants had been interviewed by clinicians about their medical history. This history included year of diagnosis for hypertension, heart disease, cerebrovascular disease, dementia, depression, Parkinson's disease, thyroid disorder, diabetes, hypercholesterolemia and cancer. The total number of physical illnesses was measured by counting the number of diagnoses for the ten chronic diseases listed above.

Depressive symptoms—A Cantonese 15-item version of the Geriatric Depression Scale (GDS) (Parmelee and Katz, 1990) was used to measure depressive symptoms. The reliability and validity of a translated version of this scale (from English to Chinese) for assessing current depressive symptoms in older populations was established in a study in Hong Kong by Chiu et al. (1994). Participants scoring eight or above were regarded as having depressive symptoms (Chiu et al., 1994).

Physical exercise—Participants had been asked whether they participated in the following types of exercise: stretching, muscle strengthening, endurance, schematic exercise, non-schematic exercise or other exercise. The total number of different types of exercise undertaken was recorded for each participant.

Results

One of the strengths of our study is in its inclusion of not one but two measures of participants' self-reported health: SRH compared with others and SRH compared to last year. This provided considerable insight about the way that individuals see the ebb and flow of their health. Although many people reported their health as "similar to others" (70.4 percent) or "similar to last year" (61.8 percent), our results show that in comparison to others, 24.2 percent of participants gave their health a positive evaluation ("better than others"), compared to only 5.4 percent who described their health as "worse than others." Relative to their own health in the previous year, however, 32.5 percent reported it to be "worse than last year," while only 5.7 percent reported it to be "better than last year." Thus, more people rated their health positively when comparing themselves to others, whereas relatively few did so when comparing their health to what it was a year earlier. This implies that while respondents may recognize their declining health, they see it as less precipitous than that of others.

Table 4.1 shows the mean values for the main variables in the study, together with standard deviations and simple correlations. A close examination of the data reveals that age is significantly related to "SRH compared to last year" ($r = 0.048$, $p < 0.05$) but not to "SRH compared to others" ($r = -0.011$, $p > 0.05$). Thus our first hypothesis, that older age will be associated with poorer SRH, is only partially supported by the data. The number of physical illnesses ($r = .095$, $p < .01$; $r = .127$, $p < .01$), depressive symptoms ($r = .152$, $p < .01$; $r = .079$, $p < .01$) and the number of exercise types ($r = -.064$, $p < .01$; $r = -.049$, $p < .05$) are each significantly related to both forms of SRH. Hence, Hypotheses 2, that the reporting of a higher degree of physical illness will be associated with poorer SRH, Hypothesis 3, that the reporting of more depressive symptoms will be associated with poorer SRH, and Hypothesis 4, that more exercise will be associated with better SRH, are all supported by our data.

We conducted a series of path analyses to complement the simple correlation analysis summarized above and to take into account conjoint and complex (direct and indirect) relationships. Path analysis is an extension of multiple regression that allows for analysis of two or more outcome variables and for inter-correlation among predictor variables. Figure 4.1 shows the coefficients for the paths proposed in the basic model.

Results for the number of physical illnesses, depressive symptoms and the number of exercises are consistent with the simple correlations reported in Table 4.1. However, age was no longer found to be significantly related to "SRH compared to last year" ($r = .01$, $p > .05$). Specifically, after controlling for the effects of the number of physical illnesses, depressive symptoms and the number of exercise types, age was no longer a significant predictor of "SRH compared to last year." Moreover, in the path analysis, age was found to be negatively related to "SRH compared to others" ($r = -.07$, $p < .01$), suggesting that older people tend to rate their health as better than others. Because age itself was not related to "SRH compared to others" ($r = -.01$, $p > .05$; see Table 4.1), we speculate that age might have a *suppression effect* in the path analysis after controlling for the number of physical illnesses, depressive symptoms and the level of exercise. A suppression effect refers

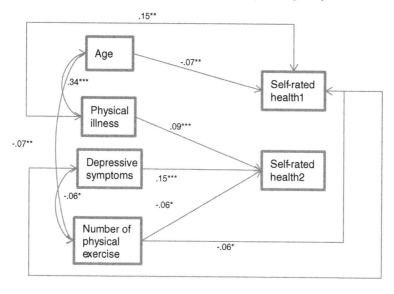

Figure 4.1 Proposed research model with path coefficients

Table 4.1 Descriptive statistics and correlations among variables

	Mean	SD	1	2	3	4	5	6
Age	74.19	5.10	1					
Number of physical illnesses	3.13	1.7	.338**	1				
Depressive symptoms	.04	.19	.013	.019	1			
Number of exercise	1.44	.71	−.070**	−.031	−.058**	1		
Self-rated health[1]	1.81	.51	−.011	.127**	.079**	−.059**	1	
Self-rated health[2]	2.27	.56	.048*	.095**	.152**	−.075**	.195**	1

Note. Only significant paths are presented.
[1] Self-rated health—compared with others;
[2] Self-rated health—compared with self last year;
* $p < .05$; ** $p < .01$.

to the inclusion of one or more predictors that suppress or remove the part of variance in a predictor that is unrelated to the outcome. Various reduced models were tested to determine the predictor(s) required to achieve the suppression effect of age. We found that when only the number of physical illnesses was included, age could have a suppression effect. In other words, once the number of physical illnesses was taken into account, age was found to be negatively related to "SRH compared to others."

Discussion

This study aimed to develop and apply a comprehensive model for describing the physical and psychological predictors of SRH in a large-scale sample of older people in Hong Kong. Overall, the findings support the four hypotheses that we generated from our review of previous studies. With respect to the simple correlations, we found that age was negatively related to "SRH compared to last year," though not to "SRH compared to others" (Hypothesis 1). Furthermore, a greater number of physical illnesses (Hypothesis 2) and depressive symptoms (Hypothesis 3), and less physical exercise (Hypothesis 4), all contributed to reporting poorer SRH defined in both comparative (to others) and longitudinal (over time) terms.

Turning to the path analysis results, while age had a weak but significant negative correlation with "SRH compared to last year," after controlling for other predictors in the path analysis, this relationship became non-significant. This loss of significance could be related to the systematic underestimation of poor health among very old individuals who may have a more limited self-awareness of their health and therefore perceive their overall health status to be better in comparison to the self-assessments of their younger counterparts with similar health conditions (Bardage et al., 2005). Similar mixed results concerning the association between age and SRH have been reported in a range of quantitative and qualitative studies (Bardage et al., 2005, Simon et al., 2005). This is suggestive of a nonlinear or curvilinear relationship between age and SRH, whereby the youngest and oldest populations tend to rate SRH positively, while middle-aged groups tend to be more negative about SRH. In one survey of elderly people, for example, the oldest individuals had the highest SRH scores (Johnson and Wolinsky, 1993). Moreover, several studies have shown that very elderly respondents tend to be more optimistic and to have diminished expectations in self-evaluations of health compared to their younger counterparts (Idler and Benyamini, 1997; Leinonen et al., 2001). Thus, observed differences may be due to aging or cohort effects (Idler, 1993). Consistent with results obtained in some previous studies conducted in Western societies, and in line with other studies on aging and health that employ Social Identity Theory, the older respondents in our study may have had diminished expectations with respect to their health and thus were more accepting of poor health in old age (Marques et al., 2015).

Our findings also suggest that objective physical illnesses and depressive symptoms can strongly and significantly predict both forms of SRH. Older adults with fewer physical illnesses and depressive symptoms tended to rate their health as "better than others" and as better than their own health in the previous year. Correspondingly, the presence of a greater number of chronic illnesses and depressive symptoms appears to contribute to a more negative SRH.

Consistent with a number of studies conducted across different cultures (Verropoulou, 2012), our results also suggest that physical and mental health conditions at baseline can predict future changes in SRH. While some studies have found that having a number of chronic conditions at baseline does not predict a decline in SRH in people aged 75 or over (Leinonen et al., 2001), our findings demonstrate a significant predictive impact of physical illnesses and depressive symptoms on SRH with increasing age, corroborating previous studies (e.g., French et al., 2012).

One important finding in this study is that physical exercise is an independent predictor of SRH. Older adults participating in regular exercise rated themselves as having better health, both compared to others and compared to themselves in the previous year. It has been demonstrated in several previous studies that physical activity can significantly decrease the risk of chronic diseases, such as cardiovascular disease and diabetes, as well as reducing other problems arising from being overweight or obese (Warburton et al., 2006). However, very few of these studies have investigated the relationship between physical exercise and self-perceived health status among older people independent of objective physical heath. Only recently has more focus been placed on studying the importance of exercise in shaping subjective health assessments in older adults and middle-aged workers (Kaleta et al., 2006; Okano et al., 2003; Ransford and Palisi, 1996).

Nevertheless, research on the effects of physical exercise on elderly people remains scarce. To the best of our knowledge, this Hong Kong study is the first to reveal the important role of physical exercise in predicting SRH in older people. The results suggest that exercise programs may hold potential for enhancing psychological well-being among older people in Hong Kong and in other jurisdictions.

The positive association between physical exercise and SRH might also be explained in terms of self-efficacy, or one's belief in one's own ability to successfully execute an action (Bandura, 1994). For example, Mullen et al. (2012) interviewed 884 community-dwelling elderly people in the United States and found that walking frequently and for a longer duration was positively related to self-efficacy, particularly as it is associated with way-finding (Mullen et al., 2012). Another randomized control exercise trial also found that self-efficacy was the most consistent determinant of physical activity among older adults (McAuley et al., 2011). Future research might focus on characterizing the underlying links between physical exercise, self-efficacy and SRH.

In terms of limitations, the main weakness of our study is its cross-sectional design. While the cross-sectional approach allowed us to include information from a larger sample, a longitudinal approach would clearly be more beneficial in future research intended to explore the causal relationships between physical/psychological predictors and SRH over a longer time period.

Another limitation was the use of medical history information that was self-reported by participants. Unfortunately, for a variety of reasons, self-reported medical history is subject to recall bias and memory error and may therefore not be a completely accurate reflection of reality.

Turning to policy implications, our results suggest that in the future, more attention should be placed on preventive programs aimed at improving subjective health through increases in physical exercise. Specifically, increasing the number and variety of physical exercise programs may increase participation. In Hong Kong, the most common forms of exercise for older adults include stretching, aerobic exercise and mind–body exercise. The latter, which includes yoga and Tai Chi, is focused on improving mental activity, relaxation and motor skills. Indeed, Tse et al. (2015) report that older people regularly involved in aerobic and mind–body exercise score higher in cognitive tests compared to their peers participating in other types of exercise. Further research exploring the effectiveness of different types of exercise in improving self-perceived health and cognitive ability would be very useful.

In conclusion, we have provided evidence of the associations between SRH and age, the presence of physical illnesses and depressive symptoms, and physical exercise. Furthermore, our findings suggest that using more than one scale to measure SRH—to capture the comparative as well as longitudinal aspects of self-assessment—holds potential for a more holistic understanding of the concept.

References

Bandura, A. (1994). *Self-efficacy*. Wiley Online Library. http://onlinelibrary.wiley.com/doi/10.1002/9780470479216.corpsy0836/full

Bardage, C., Pluijm, S.M.F., Pedersen, N.L., Deeg, D.J.H., Jylhä, M., Noale, M., Blumstein, T. and Otero, A. (2005). Self-rated health among older adults: A cross-national comparison. *European Journal of Ageing*, 2, 149–158.

Benyamini, Y., Blumstein, T., Murad, H. and Lerner-Geva, L. (2011). Changes over time from baseline poor self-rated health: For whom does poor self-rated health not predict mortality? *Psychology & Health*, 26, 1446–1462.

Canadian Institute of Health Information (2011). *Seniors and the Health Care System: What is the Impact of Multiple Chronic Condtions*. Ottawa: CIHR.

Cheng, Y., Chen, I., Chen, C.J., Burr, H. and Hasselhorn, H.M. (2013). The influence of age on the distribution of self-rated health, burnout and their associations with psychosocial work conditions. *Journal of Psychosomatic Research*, 74, 213–220.

Chiu, H.F., Lee, H.C., Wing, Y.K., Kwong, P.K., Leung, C.M. and Chung, D.W. (1994). Reliability, validity and structure of the Chinese Geriatric Depression

Scale in a Hong Kong context: A preliminary report. *Singapore Medical Journal*, *35*, 477–480.

DeSalvo, K.B., Bloser, N., Reynolds, K., He, J. and Muntner, P. (2006). Mortality prediction with a single general self-rated health question. *Journal of General Internal Medicine*, *21*, 267–275.

Falomir-Pichastor, J.M., Toscani, L. and Despointes, S.H. (2009). Determinants of flu vaccination among nurses: The effects of group identification and professional responsibility. *Applied Psychology*, *58*, 42–58.

French, D.J., Browning, C., Kendig, H., Luszcz, M.A., Saito, Y., Sargent-Cox, K. and Anstey, K.J. (2012). A simple measure with complex determinants: Investigation of the correlates of self-rated health in older men and women from three continents. *BMC Public Health*, *12*, 649.

Han, B. (2002). Depressive symptoms and self-rated health in community-dwelling older adults: Longitudinal study. *Journal of the American Geriatrics Society*, *50*, 1549–1556.

Han, B. and Jylha, M. (2006). Improvement in depressive symptoms and changes in self-rated health among community-dwelling disabled older adults. *Aging & Mental Health*, *10*, 599–605.

Haring, R., Feng, Y.S., Moock, J., Völzke, H., Dörr, M., Nauck, M., Wallaschofski, H. and Kohlmann, T. (2011). Self-perceived quality of life predicts mortality risk better than a multi-biomarker panel, but the combination of both does best. *BMC Medical Research Methodology*, *11*, 103.

Haslam, S.A., Jetten, J., Postmes, T. and Haslam, C. (2009). Social identity, health and well-being: An emerging agenda for applied psychology. *Applied Psychology*, *58*, 1–23.

Hays, J.C., Schoenfeld, D.E. and Blazer, D.G. (1996). Determinants of poor self-rated health in late life. *American Journal of Geriatric Psychiatry*, *4*, 188–196.

Heller, D.A., Ahern, F.M., Pringle, K.E. and Brown, T.V. (2009). Among older adults, the responsiveness of self-rated health to changes in Charlson comorbidity was moderated by age and baseline comorbidity. *Journal of Clinical Epidemiology*, *62*, 177–187.

Hirve, S., Oud, J.H.L., Sambhudas, S., Juvekar, S., Blomstedt, Y., Tollman, S., Wall, S. and Ng, N. (2014). Unpacking self-rated health and quality of life in older adults and elderly in India: A structural equation modelling approach. *Social Indicators Research*, *117*(1), 105–119.

Hong Kong Census and Statistics Department (2011). 2011 population census summary results. Hong Kong: Hong Kong Census and Statistics Department.

Idler, E.L. (1993). Age differences in self–assessments of health: Age changes, cohort differences, or survivorship? *Journal of Gerontology*, *48*, S289–S300.

Idler, E.L. and Benyamini, Y. (1997). Self-rated health and mortality: A review of twenty-seven community studies. *Journal of Health and Social Behavior*, *38*, 21–37.

Idler, E.L. and Kasl, S.V. (1995). Self-ratings of health: Do they also predict change in functional ability? *Journals of Gerontology, Series B: Psychological Sciences and Social Sciences*, *50*, S344–S353.

Johnson, R.J. and Wolinsky, F.D. (1993). The structure of health status among older adults: Disease, disability, functional limitation, and perceived health. *Journal of Health and Social Behavior*, *34*, 105–121.

Jones, J.M., Haslam, S.A., Jetten, J., Williams, W.H., Morris, R. and Saroyan, S. (2011). That which doesn't kill us can make us stronger (and more satisfied with life): The contribution of personal and social changes to well-being after acquired brain injury. *Psychology & Health, 26*, 353–369.

Kaleta, D., Makowiec-Dąbrowska, T., Dziankowska-Zaborszczyk, E. and Jegier, A. (2006). Physical activity and self-perceived health status. *International Journal of Occupational Medicine and Environmental Health, 19*, 61–69.

Kerr, J., Sallis, J.F., Saelens, B.E., Cain, K.L., Conway, T.L., Frank, L.D. and King, A.C. (2012). Outdoor physical activity and self rated health in older adults living in two regions of the U.S. *International Journal of Behavioral Nutrition and Physical Activity, 9*, 89. www.ncbi.nlm.nih.gov/pmc/articles/PMC3464785/pdf/1479-5868-9-89.pdf

Lee, Y. (2000). The predictive value of self assessed general, physical, and mental health on functional decline and mortality in older adults. *Journal of Epidemiology & Community Health, 54*, 123–129.

Leinonen, R., Heikkinen, E. and Jylhä, M. (2001). Predictors of decline in self-assessments of health among older people: A 5-year longitudinal study. *Social Science & Medicine, 52*, 1329–1341.

Lindström, M. (2009). Marital status, social capital, material conditions and self-rated health: A population-based study. *Health Policy, 93*, 172–179.

Marques, S., Swift, H.J., Vauclair, C.M., Lima, M.L., Bratt, C. and Abrams, D. (2015). Being old and ill across different countries: Soial status, age identification and older people's subjective health. *Psychology & Health, 30*, 699–714.

McAuley, E., Mailey, E.L., Mullen, S.P., Szabo, A.N., Wójcicki, T.R., White, S.M., Gothe, N., Olson, E.A. and Kramer, A.F. (2011). Growth trajectories of exercise self-efficacy in older adults: Influence of measures and initial status. *Health Psychology, 30*, 75.

Mullen, S.P., McAuley, E., Satariano,W.A., Kealey, M. and Prohaska, T.R. (2012). Physical activity and functional limitations in older adults: The influence of self-efficacy and functional performance. *Journals of Gerontology, Series B: Psychological Sciences and Social Sciences, 67*, 354–361.

Mulsant, B.H., Ganguli, M. and Seaberg, E.C. (1997). The relationship between self-rated health and depressive symptoms in an epidemiological sample of community-dwelling older adults. *Journal of the American Geriatrics Society, 45*, 954–958.

Okano, G., Miyake, H. and Mori, M. (2003). Leisure time physical activity as a determinant of self-perceived health and fitness in middle-aged male employees. *Journal of Occupational Health, 45*, 286–292.

Pan, X. and Ward, R. M. (2015). Diabetes self-management and self-rated health among middle-aged and older adults with type 2 diabetes in China: A structural equation model. *Social Indicators Research, 120*(1), 247–260.

Parkatti, T., Deeg, D.J.H., Bosscher, R.J. and Launer, L.L.J. (1998). Physical activity and self-rated health among 55- to 89-year-old Dutch people. *Journal of Aging and Health, 10*, 311–326.

Parmelee, P.A. and Katz, I.R. (1990). Geriatric depression scale. *Journal of the American Geriatrics Society, 38*(12).

Phillips, D.R., Siu, O.L., Yeh, A.G. and Cheng, K.H. (2005). The impacts of dwelling conditions on older persons' psychological well-being in Hong Kong: The mediating role of residential satisfaction. *Social Science & Medicine, 60*, 2785–2797.

Ransford, H.E. and Palisi, B.J. (1996). Aerobic exercise, subjective health and psychological well-being within age and gender subgroups. *Social Science & Medicine*, *42*, 1555–1559.

Segerstrom, S.C. (2013). Affect and self-rated health: A dynamic approach with older adults. *Health Psychology*, *33*, 720.

Simon, J., De Boer, J., Joung, I., Bosma, H. and Mackenbach, J. (2005). How is your health in general? A qualitative study on self-assessed health. *European Journal of Public Health*, *15*, 200–208.

Stenback, A. (1964). Physical health and physical disease as objective fact and subjective experience. *Archives of General Psychiatry*, *11*, 290.

Tajfel, H. and Turner, J.C. (1979). An integrative theory of intergroup conflict. In W.G. Austin and S. Worchel (eds), *The Social Psychology of Intergroup Relations* (pp. 23–48). Monterey, CA: Brooks/Coole.

Tran, T.V., Nguyen, D., Chan, K. and Nguyen, T.N. (2013). The association of self-rated health and lifestyle behaviors among foreign-born Chinese, Korean and Vietnamese Americans. *Quality of Life Research*, *22*, 243–252.

Tse, A.C.Y., Wong, T.W.L. and Lee, P.H. (2015). Effect of low-intensity exercise on physical and cognitive health in older adults: A systematic review. *Sports Medicine*, *1*, 1.

Verropoulou, G. (2012). Determinants of change in self-rated health among older adults in Europe: A longitudinal perspective based on SHARE data. *European Journal of Ageing*, *9*, 305–318.

Walker, J.D., Maxwell, C.J., Hogan, D.B. and Ebly, E.M. (2004). Does self-rated health predict survival in older persons with cognitive impairment? *Journal of the American Geriatrics Society*, *52*, 1895–1900.

Warburton, D.E., Nicol, C.W. and Bredin, S.S. (2006). Health benefits of physical activity: The evidence. *Canadian Medical Association Journal*, *174*, 801–809.

World Health Organization (WHO) (1990). Diet, nutrition and the prevention of chronic diseases, Geneva: World Health Organization. Report No. 797. http://apps.who.int/iris/bitstream/10665/39426/1/WHO_TRS_797_(part1).pdf.

World Health Organization (WHO) (2015). The European health report 2015, Geneva: World Health Organization. www.euro.who.int/__data/assets/pdf_file/0008/284750/EHR_High_EN_WEB.pdf?ua=1.

Zavras, D., Tsiantou, V., Pavi, E., Mylona, K. and Kyriopoulos, J. (2013). Impact of economic crisis and other demographic and socio-economic factors on self-rated health in Greece. *European Journal of Public Health*, cks143, 23(2), 206–210.

Section 2

Aging families

Caregiving and gender

5 Men providing care to aging parents in the internet age

Part of the stalled gender revolution?

Lori D. Campbell and Michael P. Carroll

Although it's long been acknowledged in the gerontological literature that most unpaid caregivers providing care to an aging parent are women, it's also been something of a convention to pair that acknowledgment with a statement indicating that things are expected to change as more and more men move into that role. Thus, Hibbard et al. (1996, p. 16) suggested that the proportion of caregivers who were male was expected to rise "as younger women are more often employed and unavailable for caregiving." In the chapter written for the 1996 collection that serves as the inspiration for this volume, it was suggested that male caregiving would rise as the result of "shrinking family size, more women employed outside the home, and greater flexibility within gender roles" (Campbell, 1996, p. 2). Clearly, then, at the turn of this century, the idea that an increase in male filial caregiving was imminent was very much "in the (scholarly) air"—and though the reasons varied somewhat from commentator to commentator, "increasing female labor force participation" and "changing gender roles" were on everyone's list.

There were, of course, some who saw a different—and bleaker—future. Frederick and Fast (1999), for example, in considering eldercare in Canada, predicted simply that with more women in the workforce and other demographic changes, there would be relatively fewer informal caregivers available—with the result that caregiver burnout, and so the need for institutionalization, would increase. Other commentators, noting the effects of globalization on world economies, and the slashing of benefits and social supports that usually accompanies globalization, foresaw that there would be an expanded demand in dual-career, middle-class households in wealthy nations for mainly female (and poorly paid) migrant workers and that a great many of these female migrant workers would take on caregiving roles. Glenn (2010), for instance, took note of the increasing reliance on paid home care workers and pointed out (using US Census data) that paid personal and home care aides were overwhelmingly women (91.8 percent), and disproportionately people of colour (49.7 percent) and immigrants (24.9 percent). The implicit prediction being made, in other words, was that while white women working full time might indeed provide less unpaid care to the elderly than previously, the slack would be taken up by poorly paid women of colour.

So, after almost two decades, what has happened in regard to male filial caregiving? Have we indeed moved closer toward the gender parity in unpaid caregiving predicted by (some) commentators? Partly, of course, the answer depends on how you measure "caregiving" and what sort of caregiving you examine. Data from the 2012 Canadian General Social Survey (GSS) suggest that the gender gap in filial caregiving has narrowed, with men making up 46 percent of filial caregivers and women the remaining 54 percent (Sinha, 2013). However, a report by the Alzheimer's Association in the US (March, 2014) indicates that women comprise 63 percent of Alzheimer's and dementia caregivers. But such numbers only tell part of the story. Paying attention to the amount of time devoted to caregiving reveals a more pronounced gender gap. The Alzheimer's Association (March, 2014), for instance, also reports that there are 2.3 times more women than men who have been providing such care for more than five years.

Further, if we agree that the most central dimensions of the caregiving role typically involve the "higher intensity" personal and domestic care tasks and responsibilities, then we find additional evidence that a significant gender imbalance in filial care continues to persist. Women continue to assume primary responsibility for care tasks that are more frequent, intense and hands-on, including personal care such as bathing and dressing, and household chores such as preparing meals; men's filial care continues to centre on tasks of financial management and home maintenance—tasks that are typically less frequent, less intense, less domestic and less personal (Sinha, 2013). Similarly, Duxbury et al. (2009, p. 32) suggest that when men do provide care, they are more likely than women to be "low intensity caregivers."

Even so, reporting the data in this way (i.e., focusing on the caregiver responsibilities assumed by women) probably diverts attention from what is likely a more significant finding, at least if our concern is with assessing the likelihood that more men will take on the caregiving role in the near future: the fact that men *avoid* these higher intensity tasks. Thus, Grigoryeva (2014) found that daughters spent more than twice the number of hours on parent care per month as sons (12.3 hours compared to 5.6 hours). The gender gap narrows a bit when other factors are taken into account, but still remains significant. The most important finding from Grigoryeva's analysis, however, is that while the amount of time that daughters devote to parent care is affected by demographic variables in ways we would expect—so that daughters employed full time (just as commentators in and since the 1990s found) do devote less care to a parent than daughters employed part-time; married women provide less care than unmarried women; daughters living at a distance provide less care than daughters living close by—this is *not* true for sons. In other words, *none* of the variables that influenced caregiving by daughters (employment status, marital status, geographical proximity) had any significant effect on levels of parental caregiving by sons. In Grigoryeva's (2014: pp. 26–27) own summary:

> These results imply that for sons, the gender norm of not doing elder care is so strong that the other factors of parent care provision essentially do not matter ... In other words, women do as much parent care as they can, given the constraints they face, while men appear to perform as little as they can, regardless of other factors.

Importantly, the pattern evident in Grigoryeva's analysis is consistent with a more general cultural pattern that has been noted by feminist authors for some time now, but that has generally been overlooked by gerontological investigators predicting a rise in male caregiving.

England (2010), for instance, starts a well-known feminist essay by acknowledging that there has undeniably been a gender revolution in a number of areas since the 1960s, and notes in particular that: women's employment has increased dramatically; women have surpassed men with regard to college graduation rates; gender discrimination in employment and education was made illegal; and women have increasingly entered many occupations previously dominated by males. Even so, she also notes that progress has been "uneven and stalled" for one simple reason: a continuing and ongoing cultural tendency to devalue activities and occupations traditionally associated with women. This is why, she argues, most occupational change in the gender revolution has involved women moving into jobs traditionally associated with men with very little movement in the opposite direction, i.e., very little movement of men into jobs traditionally associated with women (and that of course would include caregiving roles, paid or unpaid). The core point here—that the continuing devaluation of tasks traditionally associated with females has meant that "success" in the gender revolution has mainly involved females moving into traditionally male areas—has been documented cross-nationally (Charles, 2011) and is routinely included in textbooks on gender written by feminist scholars (see Wade and Ferree (2015) for a good example).

England goes on to argue that there is much evidence suggesting that a cultural emphasis on "equal rights" for men and women co-exists (however paradoxical it might seem) with a continuing belief in gender essentialism, i.e., the belief "that men and women are innately and fundamentally different in interests and skills" (England, 2010, p. 161). Glenn (2010) similarly identifies the continuing cultural belief that women are naturally better suited to caregiving as one of the conditions that "coerce" women into accepting unpaid caregiving roles. In Stacey's (2011) study of paid homecare workers, who were overwhelmingly female, she found that they typically made reference to essentialist beliefs about caregiving in justifying their own careers. Finally, Ferber (2014, p. 232) argues that this continuing belief in gender essentialism has in fact been fueled by the widespread

postfeminist belief that since women enjoy the same legal rights and opportunities as men, "any inequality between men and women, therefore, is seen
as the result of men's and women's different natures, and the choices men
and women make." Gender essentialism, then, and in particular the belief
that women are inherently more nurturing than men, seems alive and well,
notwithstanding the other gains that have undeniably been made.

Nor does the entry of some men into caregiving roles necessarily undermine this belief in gender essentialism. O'Connor's (2015, p. 202) study of
male nurses, for instance, found that while there was some evidence of a
concern for caring and nurturance among the men interviewed, they tended
to play this down in favor of an emphasis on having "fallen into nursing by
virtue of circumstance and haphazardery." In our own study of 58 men caring for an elderly parent (Campbell and Carroll, 2007), we found that most
of these male caregivers embraced the essentialist view that women were
naturally more nurturing than men and explained their own caregiving by
reference to abstract principles (e.g. "they cared for me, and so it's only fair
I care for them").

In summary, then, despite the undeniable progress that has been made in
many areas in regard to gender, the continuing and widespread belief that
women are innately more adept at providing care and nurturance, is likely
at least one of the reasons why the predicted increase in male caregivers has
been minimal at best if only because, at least in the case of informal care
(e.g. caring for an elderly parent), it (1) puts pressure on women to become
caregivers and (2) provides men with a ready-made excuse for disassociating
themselves from an activity that continues to be culturally devalued.

The larger issue here, of course, is whether cultural beliefs about gender
essentialism—which have long been under attack in public discourse—will
be sufficiently undermined over the next few years (or maybe, decades) to
make any appreciable difference in the patterns discussed above. In the
remainder of this chapter, we want to assess that issue, at least a small part
of it, by looking at something else that has generally gone unnoticed in the
gerontological literature on male caregiving: the explosive rise of the internet over the past two decades, the concomitant rise in websites directed at
people caring for an elderly parent, and what effect the advice and information presented on these websites might or might not have on attracting more
men to the caregiving role.

The rise of the internet and caregiving websites

It was only during the early 1990s that the internet, or at least what we now
recognize as the internet, first emerged in public consciousness (Streeter,
2011). This means that the internet was not really a significant presence
when *Difficult Issues in Difficult Times* (Joseph, 1996) was first published.
As every reader knows, that has changed quite dramatically. Not only are
there now countless websites in existence, with more being created every

day, but the ease of accessing these sites has been enhanced over the past decade given that they can now be accessed by using smartphones and tablets as well as personal computers. What makes all this relevant to the discussion here is that many websites that now exist are being accessed by (and addressed to) caregivers looking for help and advice.

A Pew Research Center survey (February, 2013) found that 59 percent of the respondents reported that they had gone online to seek health information in the past year; of these, 39 percent said that were looking for information on their own health; 39 percent said they were looking for information on someone else's health; and 15 percent said they were looking on behalf of both themselves and someone else. Sadavisam et al. (2013) found that 56 percent of the respondents who went online for health information reported being surrogate users of this sort. This percentage is even higher among people who identify as caregivers (i.e., someone caring for a parent or spouse, or for a child with a disability or long-term health issues). Thus, Fox and Brenner (2012) found that 67 percent of such caregivers reported that their last search for health information was on behalf of someone else. Finally, a survey of adults providing care to an adult or child with significant health issues found that 59 percent of the caregivers with internet access said that online resources had been helpful to them in providing that care, while 52 percent said that online resources had helped with their ability to cope with the stress of caregiving (Fox et al., 2013).

It seems clear, then, that family caregivers (caring for a range of family members) are now regularly accessing the internet for caregiving information, advice and support. What we want to do in the remainder of this chapter is examine some of the more popular internet sites with information and resources addressed specifically to people caring for an elderly parent to see if what's found on these sites is likely to undermine or reinforce the gender imbalance that continues to exist with regard to filial caregiving.

Selecting websites for consideration

How do adult children caring for an elderly parent go about looking for websites that might be useful to them? We don't know the answer to that for filial caregivers specifically, but the Pew Research Center survey (February, 2013) mentioned above suggests that 77 percent of the people who looked online for health information said they began simply by entering terms in a search engine such as Google, Bing or Yahoo. Only a minority (13 percent) said they started at a known website specializing in health information, and an even smaller number (2 percent) said they started at a general site such as Wikipedia or at a social network site such as Facebook (1 percent). At least in this initial exploratory study, then, it seemed reasonable to identify caregiving websites by doing what most people do in the case of health information generally, namely, start by entering a number of words and word strings into a variety of search engines.

The word strings we used were: caregiving; caregiving for the elderly; Alzheimer's caregivers; family caregivers; advice for caregivers; caring for a parent; caring for a parent with dementia; caregiving advice; caregiver websites; caregiving websites; caring for Alzheimer patient at home; family caregiver support; and advice for caregivers of dementia patients. Each of these words or word strings was put into four different search engines. Three of these (Google, Yahoo, Bing) are likely the most popular search engines currently in use, while the fourth (DuckDuckGo) is a relative newcomer whose use seems to be on the rise. Looking only at the first page of web results (in the case of each search), and excluding ads marked as such, the goal was to identify a relatively manageable set of websites that had the following characteristics:

- They provided advice to unpaid filial caregivers, even if the site also dealt with other sorts of caregiving (e.g. spousal care; care for disabled children; care for cancer patients), paid caregiving and other health related matters.
- They were websites that regularly appeared across different search engines and across different word strings.

We fully acknowledge the limitations of this methodology. As a start, using English language search terms meant that we would not detect French language caregiving websites of the sort that might routinely be accessed in Quebec. Then, too, although the word strings we used seemed to have face validity, there are almost certainly other terms that could have been used and might have produced different results. As well, since search engine results are influenced both by searcher location and any number of other factors, other investigators—across both Canada and the US—using the same words and word strings and the same search engines might well get different results.

Even so, what quickly became apparent in our searches is that certain sites did appear over and over again, across different search engines and using several different word strings. In the end, the five websites most commonly encountered were all US sites and included: Webmd.com, AARP.org (website of the AARP Foundation), Caregiver.org (the National Alliance on Caregiving's website), Alz.org (the Alzheimer's Association's website) and Caring.com. We limited ourselves to these five because there was a noticeable gap between them and the next cluster of websites encountered as a result of the "hits" produced using our search terms.

It is important to acknowledge that websites can make use of a number of strategies to ensure that they rank high in online searches and so no claim is being made here that these five websites are necessarily "the best." The point is rather that English-speaking filial caregivers in North America, whether in Canada or the US, looking for online advice, would at least come across the five sites considered here, and so these sites seem a useful starting point for assessing what caregiving websites today say (or don't say) about caregiving and gender.

Each co-author visited each of the five websites and searched each site for articles and other entries providing advice to caregivers. Only English-language material was considered (some sites, for instance, also provided material in Spanish, Mandarin and/or Hebrew). The goal was to identify themes and issues that were common across sites, with special attention being paid to material that seemed, explicitly or implicitly, to be relevant to gender (specifically the caregiver's gender).

All five sites maintained online forums where caregivers could share experiences. There is much fascinating material here, but our concern was with the information or advice that the "experts" on these sites were providing, and so these online, caregiver-originated materials were not considered in this analysis (though we plan to look at this material in a later study).

Once each of us felt that we had identified common themes across websites independently, we met to discuss our findings and jointly decide on the common themes that emerged related to gender and caregiving.

Findings

The first thing to note about caregiving websites (or at least, the section of the sites considered here devoted to caregiving), especially for those of us used to reading academic articles, is that these sites are less interested in analysis than in providing practical advice about a range of issues and queries that routinely come up during the caregiving process—and that practical advice is typically addressed to a generic and non-gendered caregiver. For example, the one topic that appears front and centre on all these sites is "caregiver stress" and it is routine to encounter discussions of caregiver stress with titles such as "10 signs of caring too much" (Caring.com), "10 symptoms of caregiver stress" (Alz. org), "6 signs of caregiver burnout" (AARP.org), etc., and the content of these discussions (which include things like: are you losing sleep?, feeling grief over a lost relationship with recipient?, getting angry over care recipient's behaviors?, etc.) seem equally addressed to all caregivers, without regard to gender. Similarly, advice on how to *avoid* caregiver stress is also common and also (typically) gender-neutral (e.g. pay attention to your own health, find help and/or a support group, learn about the services in your local community, etc.).

On the other hand, gender *is* always mentioned in one regard that is relevant to the discussion here: these sites acknowledge that most caregivers are women. The following seem typical:

> So who are these caregivers, who are tending to the health and well-being of their aging parents, spouses, and other family members while simultaneously juggling careers, children, and many other obligations? … Well, it's women who are, for the most part, America's caregivers. Between 56 and 75 percent of "informal" (i.e., unpaid) caregivers are women, according to most surveys.
>
> (Haiken, n.d. on Caring.com)

> Gender roles play a powerful role in caregiving. Women usually wind up doing the bulk of the caregiving for older relatives.
>
> (Webmd.com, 2014)

Yet here, too, as with the academic literature, this acknowledgement of the preponderance of female caregivers is sometimes paired with an optimistic statement suggesting that male caregiving is on the rise, for example:

> The gender balance shifts to close to equal participation among 18 to 49-year-old care recipients (47 percent of caregivers are male), while among the 50+ recipients, it tips to females (32 percent male, 68 percent female) … Research suggests that the number of male caregivers may be increasing and will continue to do so due to a variety of social demographic factors.
>
> (Caregiver.org, 2012)

The source cited for this particular prediction, incidentally, is Kramer and Thompson (2002) who had recited the usual litany (women's increased labor force participation; changing gender roles; geographic mobility of adult children) in order to predict that male caregiving would rise.

What's important to point out is that while the predominance of female caregivers is acknowledged, the gender imbalance in caregiving is seen as something that will just naturally self-correct over the next few years as the result of societal forces that are well under way and so, implicitly, is not something that individual caregivers need be too concerned about.

This failure to problematize the lack of gender equity in caregiving is not because these sites avoid discussing problems associated with caregiving that need to be solved. Consider Maria Shriver's *The Shriver Report: A Woman's Nation Takes on Alzheimer's* (Shriver, 2010), which is discussed not just on Alz.org (the website for the American Alzheimer's Association, which helped sponsor the report) but also on Webmd.com and AARP.org. In providing an overview of that report, Shriver (n.d. on Alz.org) begins by very forcefully remarking on the preponderance of female caregivers *and* the toll it takes on women:

> The truth is it's women who are the ones who generally do the hands-on grunt work of caregiving—cleaning their parents or spouses and changing their diapers, feeding them, babysitting them, dispensing medication to them. While men do represent about a third of family caregivers, they tend to arrange or supervise outside services.

So what's to be done? Shriver continues:

> American women are stressed-out and maxed-out. There's nothing wrong with them! They just need support. What has to get right is our institutions. They need to respond to the changing dynamic in the

American home. People with Alzheimer's cannot live alone and the family members who live with them and take care of them need help.

She goes on to list a number of changes (tax credits, flexible hours for caregivers who are employed, eldercare leave, government regulations to prevent elder abuse, more daycare programs, government support for respite programs, etc.) that would ameliorate the need for caregiver support.

Shriver is by no means the only one calling for more institutional support for caregivers. To take just one example, an entry in a report on another site issues the same call for change:

> Because of the multi-faceted role that family and informal caregivers play, they need a range of support services to remain healthy, improve their caregiving skills and remain in their caregiving role. Caregiver support services include information, assistance, counseling, respite, home modifications or assistive devices, support groups and family counseling. While many services are available through local government agencies, service organizations, or faith-based organizations, employers are beginning to implement workplace support programs as one way to mitigate the impact that caregiving can have on workers.
>
> (Caregiver.org, 2015)

We only want to call attention to what's missing: despite a recognition that women bear the bulk of the burden associated with informal caregiving and that something needs to be done about this, "getting men more involved" is not among the otherwise-numerous remedies listed.

Brothers and sisters

Threading our way through these various sites, there was one commonly encountered context where advice on getting males more involved in the filial caregiving process might reasonably have been introduced. Thus, all these sites advise filial caregivers to hold regular family discussions, and, in this context, it is common to come across concerns about equity, or really, about inequity (in other words, claims that the caregiving burden is not falling equally on all siblings). An example: "Experts say the most common source of discord among family members occurs when the burden of caring for an elder isn't distributed equally" (Matthiessen, n.d. on Caring.com).

Sometimes, gender is ignored in the advice given in these sections and caregivers are simply advised not to let old sibling relationships get in the way of making the right decisions. In other cases, however, gender is mentioned and the problem is seen to be traditional gender roles. And what do they suggest is the solution? Just set them aside, presumably as part of that erosion of gender roles that everyone knows is underway. This sentiment is reflected in the two excerpts below:

Too often, brothers expect their sisters to bear the brunt of caregiving; after all, didn't females do more family-oriented work (such as household chores) when they were all growing up together? But what woman would not fume at a brother who shirks his caregiving responsibilities today? Only when gender expectations are set aside can siblings become effective partners.

(Russo, 2011 on Caregiver.org)

Another inadvertent expectation is gender stereotyping. It's not necessarily the daughter to whom care should fall, while the son handles the money ... Remember that you're all grown-ups now, and that puts you on an equal footing. Everyone involved should have a say in what transpires.

(Scott, n.d. on Caring.com)

We would all agree, of course, that saying gender roles should be set aside is better than saying the reverse. Nevertheless, the point we want to make here is that these sites are (still) talking about gender as a role and so are ignoring the power and prestige differentials that structure and maintain gender inequalities—and which is one of the reasons why most feminist scholars set aside the "gender as role" approach decades ago (for an overview of feminist scholarship on this issue, see Ferree et al., 2007).

What is also found in these discussions about "ways for siblings to share the burden" is an emphasis on letting each sibling contribute in ways that work best for them given their preferences and abilities, as reflected in the examples below:

Many successful caregiving families report that they have divided up the responsibilities according to individual preferences and capacity. This way, everyone feels that they are contributing and the burden for the primary caregiver is significantly lightened. A family meeting can often accomplish these kinds of agreements.

(Caregiver.org, n.d.)

Divide tasks according to the family member's preferences and abilities. Some family members may be hands-on caregivers, responding immediately to issues and organizing resources. Others may be more comfortable with being told to complete specific tasks.

(Caregiver.org, n.d.)

But there's more to who is going to care for a parent than gender and age. Instead, siblings should consider who is the best fit.

(Hatfield, 2008 on Webmd.com)

The old pecking order from childhood … is ill suited to a group of caregiving adult siblings with grownup ideas, capabilities and concerns. Rather, mature sisters and brothers should work as a well-organized team in which members confer frequently, reach consensus on most decisions and divvy up tasks according to each person's talents, availability and degree of willingness.

(Jacobs, 2014 on AARP.org)

Figure out how to divide the labor. Rather than having everyone involved in every step of the care process, consider the "divide and conquer" approach. Talk over each family member's skills, strengths, and life situation.

(Scott, n.d. on Caring.com)

At one level, comments like these reflect the individualistic emphasis that pervades Western culture generally. Still, such an emphasis has a social consequence, however unintended.

Thus, as any number of commentators have noted (but see Carroll and Campbell (2008) for a literature review), it is common for men and women to "do" caregiving in different ways. Typically, commentators have suggested, male caregiving tends to be limited and instrumental, focusing on the physical well-being of the care recipient and making sure that the care recipient is happy, while female caregiving tends to be more emotionally intense and more focused on maintaining relationships. In an earlier article (Carroll and Campbell, 2008), we have already made the point that (1) the primary social function of these beliefs about "gendered styles of care" is that they can serve as scripts for caregivers to "do gender" and (2) such beliefs simultaneously serve to maintain gender inequality because it is easier to balance caregiving with ongoing full-time employment by adopting the sort of limited caregiving that is coded male than by adopting the more holistic and emotionally intense form of caregiving that is coded female.

The (additional) point we now want to make here is that although the "let everyone contribute according to their preferences and abilities" emphasis when discussing sibling contributions may not seem gendered, it is—if only because it is a perfect fit with the cultural belief just mentioned, i.e., that males and females can and should contribute to caregiving in different ways. This seems true even given (as already mentioned) the fact that these sites also advise people to put gender roles aside. Phrased differently, the "each according to their abilities and preferences" emphasis found in discussions of sibling relationships allows sons to feel at ease in restricting their caregiving activities to the sort of limited and managerial functions that typify male caregiving and so ensures that the difficult and time-consuming tasks continue to fall to daughters—and so deprives female caregivers of grounds to problematize male reluctance to take on the most time-consuming and (physically and emotionally) difficult caregiving tasks.

Summary and conclusion

In the end, then, what can we expect in regard to sons providing care to their aging parents? Predicting the future is, of course, always hazardous, and social scientists have never been particularly good at it. Still, we can examine the reasons that were adduced at by those writing at the turn of the millennium to predict a rise in male caregiving. Thus, one of those reasons was always "increasing labor force participation by women"—and we suggest it's time for commentators to recheck the data here.

Starting at the end of WW II, and for the next fifty years, the female labor force participation rate *did* increase dramatically, and this fact can rightly be considered to be one of the gender revolution's most significant successes. What is less commonly recognized in the gerontological literature, however, at least so far, is that the labor force participation rate for women appears to have peaked some time ago. In the US, this peak occurred about c. 2000 with a slight decline since (Executive Office of the President of the United States, 2014, p. 8); in Canada the participation rate for women leveled off in 2007 and then declined slightly in 2014 (Canadian Union of Public Employees, 2015; Statistics Canada, 2015). A probable cause of this leveling off/decline (in both cases) is population aging and the baby boom generation moving into retirement; even so, another contributing factor is that the female labor force participation rate for women aged 25–54 has plateaued since 2008 in both the US and Canada (Executive Office of the President of the United States, 2014, p. 35).

"Erosion of gender roles" was also regularly posited to be one of the things that would lead to more male caregiving. Here, we've already made the point, but it bears repeating, that a "gender role" approach fails to take into account gender inequalities and—in particular—the devaluation of those activities, preeminently "caring," traditionally seen as feminine. The result is that while women have moved into male areas, there has been little movement of men in the opposite direction.

In short, the optimism (and it was that) two decades ago surrounding the prediction of an imminent rise in male caregiving rested upon foundational assumptions that are now no longer true or that we can now see to be poorly conceptualized. At this point, the female labor force participation rate (which, though stable, is still high) is not likely to change dramatically, but what about the (cultural) view that "caring" is essentially feminine and devalued? Will that change? Possibly, but it does not seem to us likely in the short-term future. Certainly, while the websites examined here regularly advise their readers (at least in passing) to set gender roles aside, they do not see the continued devaluation of caregiving in the larger society to be especially problematic and so something in need of change. Indeed to the extent that these websites promote the view that "everyone should contribute according to their abilities," they are providing a definition of the situation that (however unintentionally) allows essentialist views (about women) to dictate that women, rather than men, are the ones especially well-suited to the caregiver role.

Of course, websites aside, there are other (and larger) forces making it more (not less) likely that essentialist views about female caregiving will continue to flourish. Thus, Thomas (2010) has pointed out that the continuing neoliberal de-regulation of labor markets, together with a longstanding cultural tendency for ideologies of race and gender to intersect in order to legitimize assumptions "about the 'natural' abilities of women from racialized groups" have made it even *easier* than previously to stream large numbers of women from these groups into activities such as caregiving while simultaneously continuing to devalue these activities. Thomas is talking here about paid caregivers as well as about domestic workers who clean and cook. Still, the sociological point we want to make is that by lining up racialized social categories with "women" and "caregiving" in this way, the net effect is that the cultural devaluation of caregiving in our society is sustained, not undermined.

There are many men who care for an elderly parent, and they continue to be an understudied group that deserves more attention. Still, the continuing lack of gender parity in this area must for the moment be counted as another of those areas where the gender revolution, unfortunately, seems stalled and will likely remain so for a while.

References

Alzheimer's Association. (March 2014). Women and Alzheimer's disease. *Factsheet.* Retrieved from www.alz.org/documents_custom/2014_facts_figures_fact_sheet_women.pdf.

Campbell, L.D. (1996). Caring sons: Exploring the context of caregiving. In G.M. Joseph (ed.), *Difficult issues in difficult times* (pp. 1–19). Guelph: University of Guelph.

Campbell, L.D. and Carroll, M.P. (2007). The incomplete revolution: Theorizing gender when studying men who provide care to aging parents. *Men and Masculinities*, 9(April).

Canadian Union of Public Employees (CUPE). (2015). Canada's labour force is missing something: Women. Retrieved from http://cupe.ca/canadas-labour-force-missing-something-women.

Caregiver.org. (2012). Selected caregiver statistics. Retrieved from www.bcwac.org/wp-content/uploads/2015/06/CG-Stats-from-FCA.pdf.

Caregiver.org. (2015). Women and caregiving: Facts and figures. Retrieved from https://caregiver.org/women-and-caregiving-facts-and-figures.

Caregiver.org. (n.d.). Getting sibling help with caregiving. Retrieved from https://caregiver.org/faq-more-help.

Carroll, M. and Campbell, L.D. (2008). Who now reads Parsons and Bales? Casting a critical eye on the "gendered styles of caregiving" literature. *Journal of Aging Studies*, 22, 24–31.

Charles, M. (2011). A world of difference: International trends in women's economic status. *Annnual Review of Sociology*, 37, 355–371.

Duxbury, L., Higgins, C. and Schroeder, B. (2009). Balancing paid work and caregiving responsibilities: A closer look at family caregivers in Canada. Retrieved from www.vanierinstitute.ca/include/get.php?nodeid=2382&format.

England, P. (2010). The gender revolution: Uneven and stalled. *Gender & Society*, 24(2), 149–166.

Executive Office of the President of the United States. (2014). The labor force participation rate since 2007: Causes and policy implications. Retrieved from Washington, DC: www.whitehouse.gov/sites/default/files/docs/labor_force_participation_report.pdf

Ferber, A.L. (2014). We aren't just color-blind, we are oppression blind. In M.S. Kimmel and A.L. Ferber (eds), *Privilege: A Reader* (third edn, pp. 226–239). Boulder, CO: Westview Press.

Ferree, M.M., Khan, S.R. and Morimoto, S.A. (2007). Assessing the feminist revolution: The presence and absence of gender in theory and practice. In C. Calhoun (ed.), *Sociology in America: A History* (pp. 438–479). Chicago, IL: University of Chicago Press.

Fox, S. and Brenner, J. (2012). *Family Caregivers Online*. Washington, DC: Accessed 12 July 2012, www.pewinternet.org/2012/07/12/family-caregivers-online

Fox, S., Duggan, M. and Purcell, K. (2013). *Family Caregivers are Wired for Health*. Washington, DC.

Frederick, J.A. and Fast, J.E. (1999, Autumn). Eldercare in Canada: Who does how much? *Canadian Social Trends*. Retrieved from www.statcan.gc.ca/pub/11-008-x/1999002/article/4661-eng.pdf.

Glenn, E.N. (2010). *Forced to Care: Coercion and Caregiving in America*. Cambridge, MA: Harvard University Press.

Grigoryeva, A. (2014). *When Gender Trumps Everything: The Division of Parent Care among Siblings*. Princeton, NJ: Center for the Study of Social Organizations.

Haiken, M. (n.d.). Who is a caregiver today? Retrieved from www.caring.com/articles/the-family-caregiver.

Hatfield, H. (2008). Role reversal: Caregiving for aging parents. Retrieved from www.webmd.com/healthy-aging/features/role-reversal-caregiving-for-aging-parents?page=5.

Hibbard, J., Neufeld, A. and Harrison, M. (1996). Gender different in the support networks of caregivers. *Journal of Gerontological Nursing*, 22(9), 15–23.

Jacobs, B.J. (2014). Easing age-based sibling rivalry in caregiving. Retrieved from www.aarp.org/home-family/caregiving/info-2014/caregiving-sibling-rivalry-jacobs.html?intcmp=AE-HF-IL-CRC-CAREQA.

Joseph, G.M. (ed.) (1996). *Difficult Issues in Difficult Times*. Guelph: University of Guelph.

Kramer, B.J. (2002). Introduction and purpose: Why focus on men caregivers? In B.J. Kramer and E.H. Thompson (eds), *Men as Caregivers*. Amherst, NY: Prometheus Books.

Matthiessen, C. (n.d.). Caring for elderly relatives: How to handle family conflicts. Retrieved from www.caring.com/articles/family-conflict.

O'Connor, T. (2015). Men choosing nursing: Negotiating a masculine identify in a feminine world. *Journal of Men's Studies, 23*(2), 194–211.

Pew Research Center. (February 2013). Majority of adults look online for health information. Retrieved from www.pewresearch.org/daily-number/majority-of-adults-look-online-for-health-information.

Russo, F. (2011). Caregiving with your siblings. Family Caregiver Alliance. Retrieved from www.caregiver.org/caregiving-with-your-siblings.

Sadavisam, R.S., Kinney, R.L., Lemon, S.C., Shimada, S.L., Allison, J.J. and Houston, T.K. (2013). Internet health information seeking is a team sport: Analysis of the Pew Internet Survey. *Journal of Medical Informatics, 82*, 193–200.

Scott, P.S. (n.d.). How to avoid strained sibling relationships when a parent has Alzheimer's. Retrieved from www.caring.com/articles/sibling-relationships-strained.

Shriver, M. (2010). *The Shriver Report: A Women's Nation Takes on Alzheimer's.* New York: Free Press.

Shriver, M. (n.d.). A woman's nation takes on Alzheimer's. Retrieved from www. alz.org/shriverreport/shriver.html.

Sinha, M. (2013). Portrait of caregivers, 2012. Retrieved from www.statcan.gc.ca/pub/89-652-x/89-652-x2013001-eng.htm.

Stacey, C.L. (2011). *The Caring Self: The Work Experience of Home Care Aides.* Ithaca, NY: Cornell University Press.

Statistics Canada. (2015). Employment trends of women and men aged 15 and over, 1976 to 2009. Retieved from www.statcan.gc.ca/pub/89-503-x/2010001/article/11387/tbl/tbl001-eng.htm.

Streeter, T. (2011). *The Net Effect: Romanticism, Capitalism, and the Internet.* New York: New York University Press.

Thomas, M. (2010). Neoliberalism, racialization, and the regulation of employment standards. In S. Braedley and M. Luxton (eds), *Neoliberalism and Everyday Life* (pp. 68–89). Montreal and Kingston: McGill-Queen's University Press.

Wade, L. and Ferree, M.M. (2015). *Gender: Ideas, Interactions, Institutions.* New York: W.W. Norton & Company, Inc.

Webmd.com. (2014). Finding strength as a caregiver. Retrieved from www.webmd.com/mental-health/caregiver-finding-strength.

6 Dynamic care networks

The changing face of family caregiving

Adam Davey, Maximiliane E. Szinovacz and Katherine W. Bauer

Introduction

Much of what we know about caregiving has been relatively static in nature and directed toward consideration of a single primary caregiver. More recently research, including our own, has begun to challenge this paradigm by extending caregiving theory and research in order to better understand the dynamic network context in which care most often unfolds. In this chapter, we review the current state of knowledge as it affects dynamic care networks, and present a conceptual model that can help to refine our understanding of caregiving contexts.

Caregiving is prevalent

Caregiving is increasingly prevalent, with an estimated 8 million Canadians providing care for a disabled friend or relative (Sinha, 2013). An estimated 65 million Americans provide care to a family member (National Alliance for Caregiving in collaboration with AARP, 2009), most often for a parent or parent-in-law (Wolff and Kasper, 2006), up from an estimated seven households in 1987 (Wagner, 1997). In recent years, care provided by adult children has become the most prevalent type of family care (Wolff and Kasper, 2006), but we know less about adult child caregivers and the unique stress of providing care at younger ages than spouse caregivers (Pinquart and Sörensen, 2006). Caregiving is expensive, bringing significant costs for individuals, families, and societies. The value of informal caregivers' contributions has been estimated at over $450 billion in 2009, up from $357 billion in 2007 (Feinberg et al., 2011). Caregiver costs to businesses (due to absenteeism, replacement, etc.) exceed $11 billion (Albert and Schulz, 2010). Long-term economic costs to caregivers have been documented as well. Analyses based on the Health and Retirement Study (HRS) suggest that total wage, Social Security, and pension losses due to caregiving average $303,880 for a typical caregiver (Albert and Schulz, 2010). These estimates derive from economic loss during the caregiving period and fail to consider the effect of disrupted careers on future employment.

Care is most often provided in networks

Although most caregiving research has focused on a single (primary) caregiver, our work on care networks suggests that parent care is most often shared, that care networks are dynamic, and that some networks are more enduring than others (Gaugler, 2009; Szinovacz and Davey, 2013a). Although involvement of multiple caregivers can potentially reduce the help provided by any one individual, it can also signal greater needs of the care recipient and may also require greater coordination of care and provide opportunities for conflict as a source of secondary stress (Fingerman et al., 2008; Matthews, 1987; Pillemer and Suitor, 2006).

Caregiving affects psychological and physical health

Most current caregiver research and especially interventions have focused on psychological rather than physical outcomes, and on individuals rather than networks. For this reason, we do not know how best to intervene with a care network in order to provide the most effective supports for older adults and their family caregivers. Further, effects of caregiving can be expected to have physical consequences, particularly for characteristics such as weight gain, insulin regulation, and diabetes mellitus (DM). These consequences are likely to persist well beyond the period during which care is provided and may even change an individual's set point for DM risk for a given weight status or health behaviors. Yet, we know very little about post-care experiences.

Health consequences of care persist after care stops

Studies have demonstrated reduced mental health up to five years past the care recipient's death (Aneshensel et al., 2004; Robinson-Whelan et al., 2001). Chronic stressors, such as caregiving, have been shown to affect hormonal and immunological functioning, and these effects can be seen for more than two years after caregiving responsibilities have ended (Glaser et al., 2000; Gouin et al., 2008, 2012; Kiecolt-Glaser et al., 1991; Robinson-Whelan et al., 2001; Vitaliano et al., 2003; Wu et al., 1999). Previous research using the HRS with spouse caregivers found that caregiving experiences, particularly intensive care (14+ hours/week) were associated with higher probabilities of incident hypertension (Capistrant et al., 2012a) and cardiovascular disease (Capistrant et al., 2012b), which fall along a similar pathway of inflammation. Stress leads to inflammation which, in turn, leads to atherosclerosis, insulin resistance, Type 2 DM, and metabolic syndrome, because the stress, inflammatory, and immune systems all evolve from the phagocyte (Black, 2003).

What we do not know

Research on the physical consequences of care lags behind research on psychological consequences, representing a significant knowledge gap. We know that caregiving predicts incident hypertension and cardiovascular disease among spouses, but links between caregiving and incident DM have not yet been established. We expect caregiving to predict incident DM among adult child caregivers for several reasons. Central among these are: 1) changes in weight (BMI), 2) reduced time for and engagement in vigorous physical exercise, 3) poorer health behaviors including greater rates of smoking and alcohol use, and 4) greater exposure to chronic primary and secondary stressors. With regard to the latter point, caregiving is a complex phenotype. We do not know which aspects of caregiving (e.g., care intensity, sharing of care among family members) are most strongly associated with negative health outcomes, especially from longitudinal and population-based data. Finally, 5) we know very little about post-care experiences.

Conceptual framework

Our conceptual framework (Figure 6.1) uses a life course perspective (Elder Jr., 1995; Settersten, 2003b) to expand the stress-process model (Lyons et al., 2000; Pearlin and Skaff, 1996; Pearlin et al., 1981, 1990) through

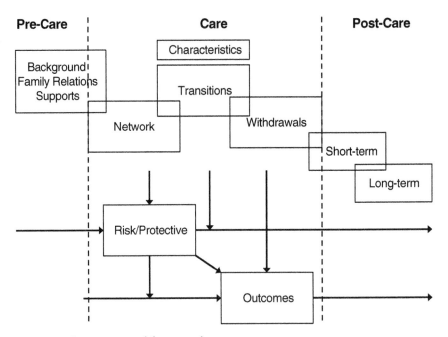

Figure 6.1 Our conceptual framework

its emphasis on long-term patterns of change in and between selected life domains. The original stress process model suggests that care outcomes (e.g., weight gain, DM) are contingent on both objective and subjective primary stressors (e.g., objective characteristics of the care situation such as care hours or care recipient's condition as well as subjective perceptions of the care situation, such as caregiver burden or role overload), secondary stressors such as work role conflict with the caregiving role or a diminished self-concept, and resources especially in the form of social supports and coping abilities. The latter are assumed to buffer stressor effects on outcomes.

The stress process model further considers background and contextual factors (gender, socioeconomic status, race/ethnicity, rural/urban residence) that may influence exposure to stressors, availability of resources, and outcomes (Aneshensel et al., 1995). Here, we outline the elements critical for elaborating the stress process model to reflect dynamic care networks. The main concepts of the life course perspective relevant for our analyses are linked life domains, linked lives, context, and trajectories (Campbell and Martin-Matthews, 2003; Franks and Stephens, 1996; Matthews and Rosner, 1988; Settersten, 2003a, 2003b; Settersten and Hägestad, 1996; Suitor and Pillemer, 1994; Szinovacz and Davey, 2004, 2008b).

Shifting the emphasis from individual caregivers toward care networks, and from a static to dynamic framework, contributes several new dimensions of the caregiving experience beyond intensity and duration considered in past studies of caregiving health effects. From a care network perspective, constructs in our model intersect in systematic ways (shown as overlap in boxes) with implications for individual health outcomes. In our model, background characteristics partially constrain possibilities for the structure of care networks. An unmarried only child, for example, can only be a sole/ primary caregiver. Daughters (especially sole daughters) in a sibling network may be more likely to assume the role of sole or primary caregiver. Network characteristics similarly constrain which transitions are possible from a given state. It is not possible to add a sibling to a care network in which all siblings are already involved.

Our previous research has suggested that network characteristics also affect transition probabilities. For example, care networks tend to shrink over time and role transitions are less likely among primary caregivers (Szinovacz and Davey, 2005a, 2008a, 2013a, 2013b). Finally, some types of care withdrawals constrain the possible transitions. Parental death and the end of need for care mark the end of care for all siblings; nursing home placement and transfer of care impose no such constraints. At least two withdrawals (nursing home placement, transfer of care) may be more or less likely as a function of care configuration. In our framework, the dynamic care experiences have implications for changes in risk and protective characteristics over time (e.g., health behaviors), as well as functioning in other life domains (e.g., work, family). In turn, these dynamic processes are expected to have implications for health outcomes over the short and long term.

Care characteristics

The stress-process model implies that objective characteristics of the care situation influence care outcomes through their impact on subjective burden. Research has also demonstrated direct effects of objective care characteristics on care outcomes. Care has more negative effects on health and mental health when it is of longer duration and intensity (Pinquart and Sörensen, 2003a; Pinquart et al., 2007) or involves care for elders suffering from dementia (Ory et al., 1999; Pinquart and Sörensen, 2003a, 2003b).

Care withdrawals

Caregivers can withdraw from care in four ways: 1) relinquishing care to another family member, 2) nursing home placement, 3) death of the care recipient, or 4) no further care needs by the care recipient. These trajectories are not necessarily mutually exclusive, and caregivers may start and end care several times both for the same care recipient as well as for different recipients (e.g., parent care followed by parent-in-law care). Research on family caregivers' experiences after placing their care recipients in a facility pertains foremost to care recipients with dementia and caregiving spouses and provides somewhat contradictory evidence. Whereas several studies indicate that stress and negative psychological as well as physical health effects subside after nursing home placement (Bond et al., 2003; Eloniemi-Sulkava et al., 2002; Gaugler et al., 2007, 2009; Gold et al., 1995; Grant et al., 2002; Gräsel, 2002; Mausbach et al., 2007), others report little change or no change in selected symptoms such as high blood pressure (Grant et al., 2002; Kramer, 2000; Schulz et al., 2004; Whitlatch et al., 1999). Several investigations attest to continued burden on caregivers after their relative is placed in a nursing home (Garity, 2006; Stone and Clements, 2009; Tornatore and Grant, 2002; Whitlatch et al., 2001; Williams et al., 2008). Better adjustment has been tied to duration of care, positive interactions with the care recipient, other nursing home residents, family and friends, and nursing staff, having planned the placement, the care recipient's adjustment to the nursing home, or the extent of caregivers' involvement after placement (Davies and Nolan, 2003; Ducharme et al., 2007; Garity, 2006; Gaugler et al., 2004, 2005; Whitlatch et al., 2001). In contrast, negative interactions with friends, staff, or the care recipient, guilt or sorrow over the placement decision, role disruption or role overload, family conflict, and uncertainty about the future undermined adaptation (Garity, 2006; Gaugler et al., 2004; Stone and Clements, 2009; Williams et al., 2008). Caregivers also felt lack of control and powerlessness and viewed the choice as forced and a failure on their part (Kellett, 1999).

Studies that consider caregiving and bereavement effects refer nearly exclusively to spouse care. Thus, very little is known about how parents' death affects former adult-child caregivers. The lack of studies relying on adult children is significant because results for spouses differ from those for adult children (Bernard and Guarnaccia, 2003; Li, 2005; Schulz et al., 2006). There are also major gaps in knowledge and understanding about differences in end of care and bereavement adjustment among diverse minority ethnic, cultural, and faith groups (Corden et al., 2008). Two theoretical models have been used in this research. One indicates that bereavement should result in relief of caregiver stress and associated effects on well-being due to the elimination of care demands and anticipatory grief prior to death. An alternative model calls for a decline in well-being after bereavement due to accumulation of care stress and subsequent difficulties in dealing with the loved one's death (Bernard and Guarnaccia, 2003; Schulz, 2009). Research (including studies on caregiving spouses' bereavement) has yielded contradictory evidence. Some studies show that caregivers fare better after bereavement (Bond et al., 2003; Keene and Prokos, 2008; Mausbach et al., 2007; Schulz et al., 1997) while others demonstrate lingering psychological and physical health symptoms (Bernard and Guarnaccia, 2003; Robinson-Whelan et al., 2001), and yet others report curvilinear relationships (Aneshensel et al., 2004; Li, 2005). Bereavement adjustment has been linked to caregiver stress prior to bereavement. Strained caregivers may be more likely to experience relief, whereas non-caregivers and less strained caregivers tend to demonstrate decreased well-being after the partner's death (Schulz and Sherwood, 2008). In one of the few studies that included adult-child caregivers, Aneshensel et al. (2004) followed caregivers who experienced bereavement sometime between the baseline interview and the last interview after five years. They found four divergent trajectories in regard to depressive symptoms: repeatedly depressed (high depressive symptoms throughout the period), temporarily distressed (depressive symptoms decline over time), repeatedly symptomatic (continuous low-level depressive symptoms), and repeatedly asymptomatic (repeatedly no depressive symptoms). The most prevalent group was repeatedly symptomatic. Repeatedly distressed caregivers tended to be female, older, lacked emotional support, and scored high on prior depressive symptoms and grief. Relationship (spouse versus adult child) did not relate to the depression trajectory. In contrast, Li (2005) reports divergent trajectories for spouse and adult-child caregivers. Wives experienced more depressive symptoms up to and shortly after bereavement followed by a steep decline in depressive symptoms about three years after bereavement, whereas daughters scored lower than wives on depressive symptoms before and up to three years after bereavement but then showed little further recovery. Because of its strong emphasis on primary caregivers and illnesses such as dementia, stroke, and cancer, the literature does not provide clear guidance regarding the effects of transferring care or resolution of care.

Risk and protective factors

Mounting evidence suggests that caregiving promotes high-risk and reduces positive health behaviors (Acton, 2002; Hoffman et al., 2012; Schulz and Sherwood, 2008). For example, compared to non-caregivers, caregivers were more likely to smoke, consume fast foods, and less likely to exercise. Such behaviors were, on the one hand, linked to stress and distress, and, on the other hand, to physical health outcomes (Hoffman et al., 2012). This trend is troubling because positive health behaviors such as exercise can decrease stress-related cardiovascular reactivity (King et al., 2002). Caregiving also has economic consequences. Caregivers, and especially caregiving women, tend to reduce their work hours (Bolin et al., 2008; Ettner, 1995; Johnson and LoSasso, 2000; Pavalko and Artis, 1997; Spiess and Schneider, 2003; Wakabayashi and Donato, 2005) and take more leave or are more absent from their jobs (Barling et al., 1994; Burton et al., 2004; Chung et al., 2008; Pavalko and Artis, 1997). They are also more likely than non-caregivers to withdraw from the labor force or opt for earlier retirement (Dentinger and Clarkberg, 2002; Ettner, 1995; Evandrou and Glaser, 2004; Pavalko and Henderson, 2006), withdrawals that are sometimes viewed as "off time" and involuntary (Szinovacz and Davey, 2005b). Such withdrawals can undermine psychological well-being (Szinovacz and Davey, 2004), especially if employment constitutes an important role and provides needed resources (Dunham and Dietz, 2003; Reid and Hardy, 1999; Rozario et al., 2004; Stephens and Townsend, 1997). Reduced work hours or leaving the labor force undermine caregivers' financial status in the long term. Together with high out-of-pocket caregiving costs, this leads to increased poverty and more reliance on government financial assistance (McDonald et al., 2000; Metlife Mature Market Institute, 2011; Wakabayashi and Donato, 2005, 2006). The familial consequences of caregiving are still not well understood. Some research indicates heightened marital conflict, lack of support from spouses, as well as conflict among family members about how to best care or how to distribute care for elder relatives (Franks and Stephens, 1996; Matthews and Rosner, 1988; Suitor and Pillemer, 1994; Szinovacz and Davey, 2008b). In addition, many caregivers face conflicts between their caregiving and other family roles and demonstrate concern that they do not do enough for their spouses or children (Dunham and Dietz, 2003; Stephens and Franks, 1995; Stephens et al., 2001), whereas caregivers' children lament lack of attention on the part of their caregiving parents (Szinovacz, 2003, 2008).

Background characteristics

The most frequently considered contexts in caregiver research include gender, race/ethnicity, socioeconomic status, and location of residence.

Research indicates that women provide more personal care than men and are given less choice in taking on care, leading to more pronounced effects of caregiving on their mental and physical health as well as their economic well-being (Canadian Study of Health and Aging, 1994; Pinquart and Sörensen, 2006; Wakabayashi and Donato, 2005, 2006; Wolff and Kasper, 2006; Yee and Schulz, 2000). However, some research suggests that male caregivers may be particularly prone to suffer physiological health effects (Zhang et al., 2006). These gender differences can be attributed to normative as well as structural factors (Campbell and Martin-Matthews, 2003; Gerstel and Gallagher, 2001; Lawrence et al., 2002; Sarkisian and Gerstel, 2004; Szinovacz and Davey, 2008a). Gender of the parent matters as well. Recipients of adult-child care are more likely to be mothers than fathers because wives tend to outlive their husbands and serve as primary caregivers for their spouses (Szinovacz and Davey, 2008a). Because same-sex caregivers are often preferred over cross-sex caregivers (Allen et al., 2012), this also promotes care by daughters rather than by sons (Szinovacz and Davey, 2008a). Studies suggest that African Americans are more involved in care but suffer fewer effects on psychological well-being than Whites (Pinquart and Sörensen, 2005; Roff et al., 2004; Skarupsky et al., 2009), although contradictory evidence has been reported as well (Lum, 2005), and outcomes may depend on whether or not caregivers live with the care recipient (Siegler et al., 2010; Skarupsky et al., 2009). African Americans' greater involvement in care can be attributed to stronger filial responsibility norms (Call et al., 1999; Dilworth-Anderson et al., 2004; Lee et al., 1998), greater cultural justification for caregiving (Janevic and Connell, 2001), less inclination to use nursing homes (Dilworth-Anderson et al., 2002; Johnson, 2008), and reduced access to high-quality institutional care (Smith et al., 2007). Similarly, Hispanic caregivers tend to view caregiving more positively than non-Hispanic Whites and tend to delay institutionalization (Coon et al., 2004; Mausbach et al., 2004; Montoro-Rodriguez and Gallagher-Thompson, 2009).

Higher socioeconomic status may protect caregivers from non-care stressors and ease their access to formal services and the healthcare system (Pinquart et al., 2007). It may also provide a basis for positive coping strategies as income and especially education are linked to mastery (Pioli, 2010). High-income caregivers also seem to recover more rapidly after bereavement, although they may experience more pre-bereavement depressive symptoms (Atienza et al., 2001). Research on the impact of rural/urban residence on caregiving has yielded contradictory results especially in regard to caregiver outcomes such as health or mental health (Byrd et al., 2011; Goins et al., 2009). However, most studies indicate that rural caregivers rely more on informal supports, whereas urban caregivers are more inclined or able to use formal and paid help (Goins et al., 2009) and have more access to secondary helpers (Chadiha et al., 2004).

Family relations and social supports

The relationship between social supports and well-being has long been rec-ognized and applied to the stress-process model of caregiving (Aneshensel et al., 1995; Krause, 2006). Numerous studies indicate that social supports can alleviate caregiver stress and well-being, although it remains unclear whether social support has direct, mediating, or moderating effects on caregiving outcomes, such as mental or physical health (Atienza et al., 2001; Au et al., 2009; Clay et al., 2008; Franks and Stephens, 1996; Kaufman et al., 2010; Koerner et al., 2007; Miller et al., 2001; Thielemann and Conner, 2009; Wilks and Croom, 2008). Some studies further suggest that social sup-port contributes to caregivers' well-being by raising their situational control (Atienza et al., 2001), self-efficacy (Au et al., 2009), or the quality of the rela-tionship between caregiver and care recipient (Chang et al., 1998). Support for caregivers can come from various sources, including spouses, siblings, friends and neighbors, as well as religious and other social groups (Koerner et al., 2007; Krause, 2002, 2006; Suitor and Pillemer, 1996; Szinovacz and Davey, 2008a, 2008b). Different support sources tend to provide divergent types of support. For example, spouses provide more emotional support, whereas siblings offer more instrumental help (Suitor and Pillemer, 1996). However, not all supports have positive outcomes (Krause, 2006). Conflict, resentment, and other negative interactions between caregivers and their supporters may undermine caregivers' well-being and add to caregiver stress (Suitor and Pillemer, 1996). While many caregivers seek out social supports, their caregiving responsibilities can also lead to "relational deprivation" as time demands of caregiving undermine opportunities to engage in social relationships (Blieszner et al., 2007).

Conclusion

Adult children have become the most common caregivers and have many years of potential excess morbidity associated with negative caregiving health outcomes, but we know less about this group than we do about spouse caregivers. A large cohort of baby boomers is now reaching the age where parent care becomes likely, making it critical to know about both the most prevalent care experiences and consequences as well as the care experi-ences that most strongly predict deleterious health consequences, including both short- and long-term, post-care outcomes.

References

Acton, G.J. (2002). Health-promoting self-care in family caregivers. *Western Journal of Nursing Research*, 24(1), 73–86.

Albert, S.M. and Schulz, R. (2010). *The MetLife Study of Working Caregivers and Employer Health Care Costs: New Insights and Innovations for Reducing Health Care Costs for Employers*. Pittsburgh, PA: Metlife Mature Market Institute.

Allen, S.M., Lima, J.C., Goldscheider, F.K. and Roy, J. (2012). Primary caregiver characteristics and transitions in community-based care. *Journals of Gerontology, Series B: Psychological Sciences and Social Sciences, 67*(3), 362–371.

Aneshensel, C.S., Botticello, A.L. and Yamamoto-Mitani, N. (2004). When caregiving ends: The course of depressive symptoms after bereavement. *Journal of Health and Social Behavior, 45*(4), 422–440.

Aneshensel, C.S., Pearlin, L.I., Mullan, J.T., Zarit, S.H. and Whitlatch, C.J. (1995). *Profiles in Caregiving: The Unexpected Career.* San Diego, CA: Academic Press.

Atienza, A.A., Collins, R. and King, A.C. (2001). The mediating effects of situational control on social support and mood following a stressor: A prospective study of dementia caregivers in their natural environments. *Journals of Gerontology, Series B: Psychological Sciences and Social Sciences, 56*(3), S129–S139. Retrieved from http://psychsoc.gerontologyjournals.org/cgi/content/abstract/56/3/S129.

Au, A., Lai, M., Lau, K., Pan, P., Lam, L., Thompson, L. and Gallagher-Thompson, D. (2009). Social support and well-being in dementia family caregivers: The mediating role of self-efficacy. *Aging & Mental Health, 13*(5), 761–768.

Barling, J., MacEwen, K.E., Kelloway, E.K. and Higginbottom, S.F. (1994). Predictors and outcomes of elder-care-based interrole conflict. *Psychology and Aging, 9*(3), 391–397.

Bernard, L. and Guarnaccia, C. (2003). Two models of caregiver strain and bereavement adjustment: A comparison of husband and daughter caregivers of breast cancer hospice patients. *The Gerontologist, 43*(6), 808–816.

Black, P.H. (2003). The inflammatory response is an integral part of the stress response: Implications for atherosclerosis, insulin resistance, type II diabetes and metabolic syndrome X. *Brain, Behavior, and Immunity, 17*(5), 350–64. Retrieved from www.ncbi.nlm.nih.gov/pubmed/12946657.

Blieszner, R., Roberto, K.A., Wilcox, K.L., Barham, E.J. and Winston, B.L. (2007). Dimensions of ambiguous loss in couples coping with mild cognitive impairment. *Family Relations, 56*, 195–208.

Bolin, K., Lindgren, B. and Lundborg, P.K. (2008). Your next of kin or your own career? Caring and working among the 50+ of Europe. *Journal of Health Economics, 27*(39), 718–738.

Bond, M.J., Clark, M.S. and Davies, S. (2003). The quality of life of spouse dementia caregivers: Changes associated with yielding to formal care and widowhood. *Social Science & Medicine, 57*(12), 2385–2395.

Burton, W.N., Chen, C., Conti, D., Pransky, G. and Edington, D.W. (2004). Caregiving for ill dependents and its association with employee health risks and productivity. *Journal of Occupational and Environmental Medicine, 46*(10), 1048–1056.

Byrd, J., Spencer, S.M. and Goins, R.T. (2011). Differences in caregiving: Does residence matter? *Journal of Applied Geronotology, 30*(4), 407–421.

Call, K.T., Finch, M.A., Huck, S.M., Kane, R.A., Burr, J.A. and Mutchler, J.E. (1999). Race and ethnic variation in norms of filial responsibility among older persons. *Journal of Marriage and the Family, 61*(3), 688–699.

Campbell, L.D. and Martin-Matthews, A. (2003). The gendered nature of men's filial care. *Journals of Gerontology, Series B: Psychological Sciences and Social Sciences, 58*(6), S350–S358.

Canadian Study of Health and Aging. (1994). Patterns of caring for people with dementia in Canada. *Canadian Journal of Aging, 13*(4), 470–487.

Capistrant, B.D., Moon, J.R. and Glymour, M.M. (2012a). Spousal caregiving and incident hypertension. *American Journal of Hypertension*, 25(4), 437–443.

Capistrant, B.D., Moon, J.R., Berkman, L.F. and Glymour, M.M. (2012b). Current and long-term spousal caregiving and onset of cardiovascular disease. *Journal of Epidemiology & Community Health*, 66(10), 951–956.

Chadiha, L.A., Morrow-Howell, N., Proctor, E.K., Picot, S.J., Gillespie, D.C., Pandey, P. and Dey, A. (2004). Involving rural, older African Americans and their female informal caregivers in research. *Journal of Aging and Health*, 16(5 Suppl), 18S–38S.

Chang, B.H., Noonan, A.E. and Tennstedt, S.L. (1998). The role of religion/ spirituality in coping with caregiving for disabled elders. *The Gerontologist*, 38(4), 463–470.

Chung, E., McLarney, C. and Gillen, M.C. (2008). Social policy recommendations to alleviate stress among informal providers of elder care. *International Journal of Sociology & Social Policy*, 28(9/10), 340–350.

Clay, O.J., Roth, D.L., Wadley, V.G. and Haley, W.E. (2008). Changes in social support and their impact on psychosocial outcome over a 5-year period of African American and white dementia caregivers. *International Journal of Geriatric Psychiatry*, 23(8), 857–862.

Coon, D.W., Rubert, M., Solano, N., Mausbach, B., Kraemer, H., Arguëlles, T., Haley, W.E., Thompson, L.W. and Gallagher-Thompson, D. (2004). Well-being, appraisal, and coping in Latina and Caucasian female dementia caregivers: Findings from the REACH study. *Aging & Mental Health*, 8(4), 330–345.

Corden, A., Hirst, M. and Nice, K. (2008). *Financial Implications of Death of a Partner*. York: University of York.

Davies, S. and Nolan, M. (2003). "Making the best of things": Relatives' experiences of decisions about care-home entry. *Ageing & Society*, 23(4), 429–450. Retrieved from http://ejournals.ebsco.com/direct.asp?ArticleID=2D7UFLC3PFBTM3MC YLL2.

Dentinger, E. and Clarkberg, M. (2002). Informal caregiving and retirement timing among men and women: Gender and caregiving relationships in late midlife. *Journal of Family Issues*, 23(7), 857–879.

Dilworth-Anderson, P., Goodwin, P.Y. and Williams, S.W. (2004). Can culture help explain the physical health effects of caregiving over time among African American caregivers? *Journals of Gerontology, Series B: Psychological Sciences and Social Sciences*, 59(3), S138–145.

Dilworth-Anderson, P., Williams, I.C. and Gibson, B.E. (2002). Issues of race, ethnicity and culture in caregiving research: A 20-year review (1980–2000). *The Gerontologist*, 42(2), 237–272. Retrieved from http://gerontologist. gerontologyjournals.org/cgi/content/abstract/42/2/237.

Ducharme, F., Levesque, L., Lachance, L., Gangbe, M., Zarit, S., Vezina, J. and Caron, C. (2007). Older husbands as caregivers: Factors associated with health and the intention to end home caregiving. *Research on Aging*, 29, 3–31.

Dunham, C. and Dietz, B. (2003). "If I'm not allowed to put my family first": Challenges experienced by women who are caregiving for family members with dementia. *Journal of Women and Aging*, 25(1), 55–69.

Elder Jr., G. (1995). The life course paradigm: Social change and individual development. In P. Moen, J.G. Elder and K. Lüscher (eds), *Examining Lives in*

Context: Perspectives on the Ecology of Human Development (pp. 101–140). Washington, DC: American Psychological Association.

Eloniemi-Sulkava, U., Rahkonen, T., Suihkonen, M., Halonen, P., Hentinen M. and Sulkava, R. (2002). Emotional reactions and life changes of caregivers of demented patients when home caregiving ends. *Journal of Aging & Mental Health*, 6(4), 343–349.

Ettner, S.L. (1995). The impact of "parent care" on female labor supply decisions. *Demography*, 32, 63–80.

Evandrou, M. and Glaser, K. (2004). Family, work and quality of life: Changing economic and social roles throughout the lifecourse. *Ageing & Society*, 24(5), 771–791.

Feinberg, L., Reinhard, S., Houser, A. and Choula, R. (2011). Valuing the invaluable: 2011 update the growing contributions and costs of family caregiving. Retrieved from http://scholar.google.com/scholar?hl=en&btnG=Search&q=intitle:Valuing +the+Invaluable:+2011+Update+-+The+Growing+Contributions+and+Costs+of +Family+Caregiving#0.

Fingerman, K.L., Pitzer, L., Lefkowitz, E.S., Birditt, K.S. and Mroczek, D. (2008). Ambivalent relationship qualities between adults and their parents: Implications for the well-being of both parties. *Journals of Gerontology, Series B: Psychological Sciences and Social Sciences*, 63(6), P362–P371.

Franks, M.M. and Stephens, A.P. (1996). Social support in the context of caregiving: Husbands' provision of support to wives involved in parent care. *Journals of Gerontology, Series B: Psychological Sciences and Social Sciences*, 51(1), P43–P52. Retrieved from http://psychsocgerontology.oxfordjournals.org/ content/51B/1/P43.full.pdf.

Garity, J. (2006). Caring for a family member with Alzheimer's Disease: Coping with caregiver burden post-nursing home placement. *Journal of Gerontological Nursing*, 32(6), 39–48.

Gaugler, J.E. (2009), Caregiving contexts: Cultural, familial, and societal implications. *Journal of Marriage and Family*, 71, 205–207.

Gaugler, J.E., Anderson, K.A., Zarit, J.M. and Pearlin, L.I. (2004). Family involvement in nursing homes: Effects on stress and well-being. *Aging & Mental Health*, 8(1), 65–75.

Gaugler, J.E., Kane, R.L., Kane, R.A., Clay, T. and Newcomer, R.C. (2005). The effects of duration of caregiving on institutionalization. *The Gerontologist*, 45(1), 78–89.

Gaugler, J.E., Mittelman, M., Hepburn, K. and Newcomer, R. (2009). Predictors of change in caregiver burden and depressive symptoms following nursing home admission. *Psycholgy and Aging*, 24(2), 385–396.

Gaugler, J.E., Pot, A.M. and Zarit, S.H. (2007). Long-term adaptation to institutionalization in dementia caregivers. *The Gerontologist*, 47(6), 730–740.

Gerstel, N. and Gallagher, S.K. (2001). Men's caregiving: Gender and the contingent character of care. *Gender and Society*, 15(2), 197–217.

Glaser, R., Sheridan, J., Malarkey, W.B., MacCallum, R.C. and Kiecolt-Glaser, J.K. (2000). Chronic stress modulates the immune response to a pneumococcal pneumonia vaccine. *Psychosomatic Medicine*, 62(6), 804–807.

Goins, R.T., Spencer, S.M. and Byrd, J.C. (2009). Research on rural caregiving: A literature review. *Journal of Applied Geronotology*, 28(2), 139–170.

Gold, D.P., Reis, M., Markiewicz, D. and Andres, D. (1995). When home caregiving ends: A longitudinal study of outcomes for caregivers of relatives with dementia. *Journal of the American Geriatrics Society, 43*(6), 10–16.

Gouin, J.P., Glaser, R., Malarkey, W.B., Beversdorf, D. and Kiecolt-Glaser, J. (2012). Chronic stress, daily stressors, and circulating inflammatory markers. *Health Psychology, 31*(2), 264–268.

Gouin, J.P., Hantsoo, L. and Kiecolt-Glaser, J.K. (2008). Immune dysregulation and chronic stress among older adults: A review. *Neuroimmunomodulation, 15*(4–6), 251–259.

Grant, I., Adler, K., Patterson, T., Dimsdale, J., Ziegler, M. and Irwin, M. (2002). Health consequences of Alzheimer's caregiving transitions: Effects of placement and bereavement. *Pyschosomatic Medicine, 64*(3), 477–486.

Gräsel, E. (2002). When home care ends: Changes in the physical health of informal caregivers caring for dementia patients: A longitudinal study. *Journal of the American Geriatrics Society, 50*(5), 843–849.

Hoffman, G.J., Lee, J. and Mendez-Luck, C.A. (2012). Health behaviors among baby boomer informal caregivers. *The Gerontologist, 52*(2), 219–230.

Janevic, M.R. and Connell, C.M. (2001). Racial, ethnic, and cultural differences in the dementia caregiving experience: Recent findings. *The Gerontologist, 41*(3), 334–347. Retrieved from http://gerontologist.gerontologyjournals.org/cgi/content/abstract/41/3/334.

Johnson, R.W. (2008). Choosing between paid elder care and unpaid help from adult children. In M.E. Szinovacz and A. Davey (eds), *Caregiving Contexts: Cultural, Familial and Societal Implications* (pp. 35–69). New York: Springer.

Johnson, R.W. and LoSasso, A.T. (2000). *Parental Care at Midlife: Balancing Work and Family Responsibilities Near Retirement*. Washington, DC: Urban Insititue.

Kaufman, A.V., Kosberg, J.I., Leeper, J.D. and Tang, M. (2010). Social support, caregiver burden, and life satisfaction in a sample of rural African American and white caregivers of older persons with dementia. *Gerontological Social Work, 53*(3) 251–269.

Keene, J.R. and Prokos, A.J. (2008). Widowhood and the end of spousal care-giving: Relief or wear and tear? *Ageing & Society, 28*, 551–570.

Kellett, U. (1999). Transition in care: Family carers' experience of nursing home placement. *Journal of Advanced Nursing, 29*(6), 1474–1481.

Kiecolt-Glaser, J.K., Dura, J.R., Speicher, C.E., Trask, J. and Glaser, R. (1991). Spousal caregivers of dementia victims: Longitudinal changes in immunity and health. *Psychocomatic Medicine, 53*, 345–362.

King, A.C., Baumann, K., O'Sullivan, P., Wilcox, S. and Castro, C. (2002). Effects of moderate intensity exercise on physiological, behavioral, and emotional responses to family caregiving: A randomized controlled trial. *Journals of Gerontology, Series A: Biological Sciences and Medical Sciences, 57*(1), M26–36. Retrieved from http://biomed.gerontologyjournals.org/cgi/content/abstract/57/1/M26.

Koerner, S.S., Kenyon, D.B. and Shirai, Y. (2007). Caregiving for elder relatives: Which caregivers experience personal benefits/gains? *Archives of Gerontology & Geriatrics, 48*(2), 238–245.

Kramer, B.J. (2000). Husbands caring for wives with dementia: A longitudinal study of continuity and change. *Health and Social Work, 25*(2), 97–107.

Krause, N. (2002). Church-based social support and health in old age: Exploring variations by race. *Journals of Gerontology, Series A: Biological Sciences and Medical Sciences*, 57(6), S332–347. Retrieved from http://psychsoc. gerontologyjournals.org/cgi/content/abstract/57/6/S332.

Krause, N. (2006). Social relationships in later life. In R.H. Binstock and L.K. George (eds), *Handbook of Aging and the Social Sciences* (pp. 181–200). Amsterdam: Academic Press.

Lawrence, J.A., Goodnow, J.J., Woods, K. and Karantzas, G. (2002). Distribution of cargiving tasks among family members: The place of gender and availability. *Journal of Family Psychology*, 16(4), 493–509.

Lee, G.R., Peek, C.W. and Coward, R.T. (1998). Race differences in filial responsibility expectations among older parents. *Journal of Marriage and the Family*, 60, 404–412.

Li, L.W. (2005). From caregiving to bereavement: Trajectories of depressive symptoms among wife and daughter caregivers. *Journals of Gerontology, Series B: Psychological Sciences and Social Sciences*, 60B(4), P190–P198.

Lum, T. (2005). Understanding the racial and ethnic differences in caregiving arrangements. *Journal of Gerontological Social Work*, 45(4), 3–21.

Lyons, K.S., Zarit, S.H. and Townsend, A.L. (2000). Families and formal service usage: Stability and change in patterns of interface. *Aging & Mental Health*, 4(3), 234–243.

Matthews, S.H. (1987). Provision of care to old parents: Division of responsibility among children. *Research on Aging*, 9(1), 45–60.

Matthews, S.H. and Rosner, T.T. (1988). Shared filial responsibility: The family as primary caregiver. *Journal of Marriage and the Family*, 50, 185–195.

Mausbach, B.T., Aschbacher, K., Patterson, T.L., von Kanel, R., Dimsdale, J.E. and Mills, P.J. (2007). Effects of placement and bereavement on psychological well-being and cardiovascular risk in Alzheimer's caregivers: A longitudinal analysis. *Journal of Psychosomatic Research*, 62(4), 439–445.

Mausbach, B.T., Coon, D.W., Depp, C., Rabinowitz, Y.G., Wilson-Arias, E., Kraemer, H.C., Thompson, L.W., Lane, G. and Gallagher-Thompson, D. (2004). Ethnicity and time to institutionalization of dementia patients: A comparison of latina and Caucasian female family caregivers. *Journal of the American Geriatric Society*, 52, 1077–1084.

McDonald, L., Donahue, P. and Marshall, V. (2000). The economic consequences of unexpected early retirement. In F.T. Denton, D. Fretz and B.G. Spencer (eds), *Independence and Economic Security in Old Age* (pp. 267–292). Vancouver: UBC Press.

Metlife Mature Market Institute. (2011). The MetLife study of caregiving costs to working caregivers. Retrieved from www.caregiving.org/wp-content/ uploads/2011/06/mmi-caregiving-costs-working-caregivers.pdf.

Miller, B., Townsend, A., Carpenter, E., Montgomery, R.V.J., Stull, D. and Young, R.F. (2001). Social support and caregiver distress: A replication analysis. *Journals of Gerontology, Series B: Psychological Sciences and Social Sciences*, 56(4), S249–S256. Retrieved from http://psychsoc.gerontologyjournals.org/cgi/content/ abstract/56/4/S249.

Montoro-Rodriguez, J. and Gallagher-Thompson, D. (2009). The role of resources and appraisals in predicting burden among Latina and non-Hispanic white female caregivers: A test of an expanded socio-cultural model of stress and coping. *Aging & Mental Health*, 13(5), 648–658.

National Alliance for Caregiving in collaboration with AARP (2009, November). Caregiving in the US. Retrieved from www.caregiving.org/data/Caregiving_in_the_US_2009_full_report.pdf.

Ory, M.G., Hoffman III, R.R., Yee, J.L., Tennstedt, S. and Schulz, R. (1999). Prevalence and impact of caregiving: A detailed comparison between dementia and nondementia caregivers. *The Gerontologist, 39*(2), 177–185. Retrieved from http://gerontologist.gerontologyjournals.org/cgi/content/abstract/39/2/177.

Pavalko, E.K. and Artis, J.E. (1997). Women's caregiving and paid work: Causal relationships in late midlife. *Journals of Gerontology, Series B: Psychological Sciences and Social Sciences, 52*, S170–S1789.

Pavalko, E.K. and Henderson, K.A. (2006). Combining care work and paid work: Do workplace policies make a difference? *Research on Aging, 28*, 359–374.

Pearlin, L.I. and Skaff, M.M. (1996). Stress and the life course: A paradigmatic alliance. *The Gerontologist, 36*, 239–247.

Pearlin, L.I., Mullan, J.T., Semple, S.J. and Skaff, M.M. (1990). Caregiving and the stress process: An overview of concepts and their measures. *The Gerontologist, 30*(5), 583–594. Retrieved from http://gerontologist.gerontologyjournals.org/cgi/content/abstract/30/5/583.

Pearlin, L.M.A., Menaghan, I., Lieberman, E.G. and Mullan, J.T. (1981). The stress process. *Journal of Health and Social Behavior, 22*, 337–356.

Pillemer, K. and Suitor, J.J. (2006). Making choices: A within-family study of caregiver selection. *The Gerontologist, 46*(4), 439–448.

Pinquart, M. and Sörensen, S. (2003a). Associations of stressors and uplifts of caregiving with caregiver burden and depressive mood: A meta-analysis. *Journals of Gerontology, Series B: Psychological Sciences and Social Sciences, 58*(2), 112–128.

Pinquart, M. and Sörensen, S. (2003b). Differences between caregivers and noncaregivers in psychological health and physical health: A meta-analysis. *Psychology and Aging, 18*(2), 250–267.

Pinquart, M. and Sörensen, S. (2005). Ethnic differences in stressors, resources, and psychological outcome of family caregiving: A meta-analysis. *The Gerontologist, 45*(1), 90–106.

Pinquart, M. and Sörensen, S. (2006). Gender differences in caregiver stressor, social resources, and health: An updated meta-analysis. *Journals of Gerontology, Series B: Psychological Sciences and Social Sciences, 61*(1), 33–45.

Pinquart, M., Sörensen, S. and So, S. (2007). Correlates of physical health of informal caregivers: A meta-analysis. *Journals of Gerontology, Series B: Psychological Sciences and Social Sciences, 62*(2), P126–P137.

Pioli, M.F. (2010). Global and caregiving mastery as moderators in the caregiving stress process. *Aging & Mental Health, 14*(5), 603–612.

Reid, J. and Hardy, M. (1999). Multiple roles and well-being among midlife women: Testing role strain and role enhancement theories. *Journals of Gerontology, Series B: Psychological Sciences and Social Sciences, 54*(6), S329–S338. Retrieved from http://psychsocgerontology.oxfordjournals.org/content/54B/6/S329.full.pdf.

Robinson-Whelan, S., Tada, Y., MacCallum, R. and Kiecolt-Glaser, J. (2001). Long-term caregiving: What happens when it ends? *Journal of Abnormal Psychology, 110*(4), 573–584.

Roff, L.L., Burgio, L.D., Gitlin, L., Nicola, E., Chaplin, W., Hardin, J.M. and Nichols, L. (2004). Positive aspects of Alzheimer's caregiving: The role of race.

Journals of Gerontology, Series B: Psychological Sciences and Social Sciences, 59(4), P185–190.

Rozario, P., Morrow-Howell, N. and Hinterlong, J. (2004). Role enhancement or role strain: Assessing the impact of multiple productive roles on older caregiver well-being. *Research on Aging*, 26(4), 413–428.

Sarkisian, N. and Gerstel, N. (2004). Explaining the gender gap in help to parents: The importance of employment. *Journal of Marriage and Family*, 66(2), 431–451. Retrieved from www.jstor.org/stable/3599847?seq=1#page_scan_tab_contents.

Schulz, R. (2009). Caregiving, bereavement and complicated grief. *Bereave Care*, 28(3), 10–13.

Schulz, R. and Sherwood, P.R. (2008). Physical and mental health effects of family caregiving. *American Journal of Nursing*, 108(9), 23–27.

Schulz, R., Boerner, K., Shear, K., Zhang, S. and Gitlin, L. (2006). Predictors of complicated grief among dementia caregivers: A prospective study of bereavement. *American Journal of Geriatric Psychology*, 14, 650–658.

Schulz, R., Newsom, J., Fleissner, K., Decamp, A. and Nieboer, A. (1997). The effects of bereavement after family caregiving. *Aging & Mental Health*, 1(3), 269–282.

Schulz, R., Belle, S.H., Czaja, S.J., McGinnis, K.A., Stevens, A. and Zhang, S. (2004). Long-term care placement of dementia patients and caregiver health and well-being. *Journal of the American Medical Association*, 292(8), 961–967.

Settersten, R.A. (2003a). Invitation to the life course: The promise. In R.A. Settersten (ed.), *Invitation to the Life Course: Toward New Understanding of Later Life* (pp. 1–12). Amityville, NY: Baywood.

Settersten, R.A. (2003b). Propositions and controversies in life-course scholarship. In R.A. Settersten (ed.), *Invitation to the Life Course: Toward New Understanding of Later Life* (pp. 15–48). Amittyville, NY: Baywood.

Settersten, R.A. and Hägestad, G.O. (1996). What's the latest? II. Cultural age deadlines for educational and work transition. *The Gerontologist*, 36(5), 602–613.

Siegler, I.C., Brummett, B.H., Williams, R.B., Haney, T.H. and Dilworth-Anderson, P. (2010). Caregiving, residence, race, and depressive symptoms. *Aging & Mental Health*, 14(7), 771–778.

Sinha, M. (2013). Spotlight on Canadians: Results from the general social survey – portrait of caregivers 2012. *Statistics Canada*, 89, 1–21.

Skarupsky, K.A., McCann, J.J., Bienias, J.L. and Evans, D.A. (2009). Race differences in emotional adaptation of family caregivers. *Aging & Mental Health*, 13(5), 715–724.

Smith, D.B., Feng, Z., Fennell, M.L., Zinn, J.S. and Mor, V. (2007). Separate and unequal: Racial segregation and disparities in quality across US nursing homes. *HealthAffairs*, 26(5), 1448–1458.

Spiess, C.K. and Schneider, U. (2003). Interactions between care-giving and paid work hours among European midlife women, 1994 to 1996. *Ageing & Society*, 23, 41–68.

Stephens, M.A.P. and Franks, M.M. (1995). Spillover between daughter's roles as caregiver and wife: Interference or enhancement? *Journals of Gerontology, Series B: Psychological Sciences and Social Sciences*, 50, P9–P17.

Stephens, M.A.P. and Townsend, A.L. (1997). Stress of parent care: Positive and negative effects of women's other roles. *Psychology and Aging, 12*, 376–386.

Stephens, M.A.P., Townsend, A.L., Martire, L.M., Druley, J.A., Ann, M. and Stephens, P. (2001). Balancing parent care with other roles: Interrole conflict of adult daughter aregivers. *Journals of Gerontology, Series B: Psychological Sciences and Social Sciences, 56*(1), P24–P34. Retrieved from http://psychsoc. gerontologyjournals.org/cgi/content/abstract/56/1/P24.

Stone, L.J. and Clements, J.A. (2009). The effects of nursing home placement on the perceived levels of caregiver burden. *Journal of Gerontological Social Work, 52*(3), 193–214.

Suitor, J.J. and Pillemer, K. (1994). Family caregiving and marital satisfaction: Findings from a 1-year panel study of women caring for parents with dementia. *Journal of Marriage and the Family, 56*, 681–690.

Suitor, J.J. and Pillemer, K. (1996). Sources of support and interpersonal stress in the networks of married caregiving daughters: Findings from a 2-year longitudinal study. *Journals of Gerontology, Series B: Psychological Sciences and Social Sciences, 51*(6), S297–S306. Retrieved from http://psychsocgerontology. oxfordjournals.org/content/51B/6/S297.full.pdf.

Szinovacz, M.E. (2003). Dealing with dementia: Perspectives of caregivers' children. *Journal of Aging Studies, 17*, 445–472.

Szinovacz, M.E. (2008). Children in caregiving families. In M.E. Szinovacz and A. Davey (eds), *Caregiving Contexts: Cultural, Familial, and Societal Implications* (pp. 161–190). New York: Springer.

Szinovacz, M.E. and Davey, A. (2004). Retirement transitions and spouse disability: Effects on depressive symptoms. *Journals of Gerontology, Series B: Psychological Sciences and Social Sciences, 59*(6), 233–245.

Szinovacz, M.E. and Davey, A. (2005). *Changes in Adult-child Caregiver Networks*. Paper presented at the meeting of the Gerontological Society of America, Washington, DC.

Szinovacz, M.E. and Davey, A. (2005). Predictors of perceptions of involuntary retirement. *The Gerontologist, 45*(1), 36–47.

Szinovacz, M.E. and Davey, A. (2008a). Division of care among adult children. *Caregiving Contexts: Cultural, Familial and Societal Implications, 28*(4), 133–159.

Szinovacz, M.E. and Davey, A. (2008b). The division of parent care between spouses. *Ageing & Society, 28*(4), 571–597.

Szinovacz, M.E. and Davey, A. (2013a). Prevalence and predictors of change in adult-child primary caregivers. *International Journal of Aging and Human Development, 76*(3), 227–49.

Szinovacz, M.E. and Davey, A. (2013b). Changes in adult children's participation in parent care. *Ageing & Society, 33*(4), 667–697.

Thielemann, P.A. and Conner, N. (2009). Social support as mediator of depression in caregivers of patients with end-stage disease. *Journal of Hospive & Palliative Nursing, 11*(2), 82–90.

Tornatore, J.B. and Grant, L.A. (2002). Burden among family caregivers of persons with Alzheimer's disease in nursing homes. *The Gerontologist, 42*(4), 497–506. Retrieved from http://gerontologist.gerontologyjournals.org/cgi/content/ abstract/42/4/497.

Vitaliano, P.P., Zhang, J. and Scanlon, J. (2003). Is caregiving hazardous to one's health? A meta-analysis. *Psychological Bulletin, 129*(6), 946–972.

Wagner, D.L. (1997). *Comparative Analysis of Caregiver Data for Caregivers to The Elderly 1987 and 1997.* Bethesda, MD: National Alliance for Caregiving.

Wakabayashi, C. and Donato, K.M. (2005). The consequences of caring: Effects of women's employment and earnings. *Population Research and Policy Review, 24,* 467–488.

Wakabayashi, C. and Donato, K.M. (2006). Does caregiving increase poverty among women in later life? Evidence from the health and retirement survey. *Journal of Health and Social Behavior, 47,* 258–274.

Whitlatch, C.J., Feinberg, L. and Stevens, E. (1999). Predictors of institutionalization for persons with Alzheimer's disease and the impact of family caregivers. *Journal of Mental Health and Aging, 5*(3), 275–288.

Whitlatch, C.J., Schur, D., Noelker, L.S., Ejaz, F.K. and Looman, W.J. (2001). The stress process of family caregiving in institutional settings. *The Gerontologist, 41*(4), 462–473. Retrieved from http://gerontologist.gerontologyjournals.org/cgi/content/abstract/41/4/462.

Wilks, E.S. and Croom, B. (2008). Perceived stress and resilience in Alzheimer's disease caregivers: Testing moderation and mediation models of social support. *Aging & Mental Health, 12*(3), 357–365.

Williams, S.W., Desai, T., Rurka, J.T. and Mutran, E.J. (2008). Predictors of satisfaction for African-American and white family caregivers of adult care home residents. *Journal of Applied Gerontology, 27,* 568–587.

Wolff, J.L. and Kasper, J.D. (2006). Caregivers of frail elders: Updating a national profile. *The Gerontologist, 46*(3), 344–356.

Wu, H., Wang, J., Cacioppo, J.T., Glaser, R., Kiecolt-Glaser, J.K. and Malarkey, W.B. (1999). Chronic stress associated with spousal caregiving of patients with Alzheimer's dementia is associated with downregulation of B-lymphocyte GH mRNA.J. *Journals of Gerontology, Series A: Biological Sciences and Medical Sciences, 54*(4), M212–215. Retrieved from http://biomed.gerontologyjournals.org/cgi/content/abstract/54/4/M212.

Yee, J.L. and Schulz, R. (2000). Gender differences in psychiatric morbidity among family caregivers: A review and analysis. *The Gerontologist, 40*(2), 147–164. Retrieved from http://gerontologist.gerontologyjournals.org/cgi/content/abstract/40/2/147.

Zhang, J., Vitaliano, P. and Lin, H.J. (2006). Relations of caregiving stress and health depend on the health indicators used and gender. *International Journal of Behavioral Medicine, 13*(2), 173–181.

7 Revised perspective on the communication predicament between adult children and their aging parents

Valerie Powell

As a graduate student in the 1990s studying gerontology, I argued that there was a communication predicament between adult children and their aging parents (Powell, 1996). Research at that time described multiple stereotypes contributing to both positive and negative attitudes toward older people. This clash of attitudes, when trying to achieve the balance between respect and caring, can create a communication predicament between older parents and their adult children (Hummert et al., 1994; Ryan et al., 1995). Twenty years, and many lessons, later I return to the topic to explore newer insights on the communication predicament.

More recently, the concept of "ambiguity" has been introduced into the research on conflict in parent–child relationships. As a new cohort of seniors emerges, and in an ever-changing social, economic and political global environment, key questions emerge: how do stereotypes shape the communication predicament between adult children and their aging parents, and how does intergenerational ambiguity mediate family conflict that may result?

Demographic changes such as increasing longevity, declining fertility rates and falling death rates resulting from improvements in the health of older adults over the past two decades have had a significant impact on the parent–child relationship, which is one of the most long lasting and emotionally intense social ties in most peoples' lives (Birdittet al., 2009; Ontario Human Rights Commission, n.d.).

In 1996, I proposed that the Communication Predicament of Aging Model was an effective theoretical approach for understanding parent/adult child communication (Powell, 1996). This conceptual framework was initially developed to explore how age-related stereotypes lead to patronizing problematic speech, usually directed from young to old (Ryan et al., 1986). The model describes both appropriate and inappropriate modifications in communication, and the conflict between caring and nurturing. Within families, this can be described as frustration and stress versus affection and obligation (Powell, 1996). Communication between the adult child caregiver and the aging parent can affect the health and well-being of both care provider and recipient (Harwood et al., 2013). It is therefore important to explore family communication in more detail, not only to better understand *how* it shapes well-being, but also to construct a foundation upon which to build strategies that can facilitate positive interaction and transitions for the aging family.

Communication in general has been described as "ambiguous, imprecise and inherently flawed" (Williams and Nussbaum, 2001, Page ix). Moreover, communication challenges between adult children and their aging parents, particularly about transitions associated with dependency and health, have often been attributed to differing cohort experiences, assumptions about aging itself and lifestyle preferences (Williams and Nussbaum, 2001). It has been suggested that frailty of older parents and their dependence on children, if and when it occurs, can introduce friction and strain into inter-generational relationships (Silverstein et al., 2010).

In the course of my work with seniors and their families over the past 20 years, as a psychogeriatric consultant and administrator in the public sector, in my role as a Canadian federal party seniors' critic and advisor on poli-cies, and as a mother of now adult children, I have observed an increasing complexity in the issues associated with parent/adult child communication. For example, macro-contextual factors such as the economy, culture and government policy appear to have a growing and more complex influence on family relationships at the micro-level. The notion of family has become more diverse, with blended and step-family relationships, single moms or dads, remarriages and gender preferences each having an effect on care sup-port and parent/adult child relationships. In our modern era, technology also adds a new dimension to family communication. People now have the opportunity to communicate and maintain relationships electronically at a distance through texting, e-mail and personal video. As our world becomes increasingly complex, so too do the influences that shape intergenerational communication.

This chapter will begin by discussing stereotypes that affect family com-munication at the micro/individual level. The next section highlights how stereotypes incorporated into policy might also influence intergenerational communication. The third section introduces Ambiguity Theory and its mediating relationship in family conflict. The conclusion draws the discus-sion together and offers recommendations for policy and practice.

Stereotypes: the micro gaze

The term "ageism," attributed to Gerontologist and Psychiatrist Robert Neil Butler, is defined as "a process of systematic stereotyping or discrimination against people because they are old" (Cruikshank, 2013, p. 136). Ageism is perpetuated through a process of internalized stereotypes about aging that begins in childhood and continues through adult life (Levy, 2009). Some of these stereotypes come from personal experiences that become over-generalized. For example, Keaton and Giles (2015) found that university students often avoided interacting with older adults because they expected older peoples' conversations to be off topic, provide too much information and to be excessive, making younger people feel uncomfortable. In another study, Bodner et al. (2012) found that middle-aged adults, the age group predominantly involved in parent–adult child communication about eldercare, expressed more ageist views than members of both younger and older groups, particularly in their views about older adults' lack of contribution to society.

In a study of adult children and their imagined conversations with aging parents about future care needs, Pitts et al. (2014) used measures associated with an older adult's positive or negative "face" upon receiving the message. Positive face was based upon the speaker communicating attributes and accomplishments (such as competence, selflessness and independence) of her/his parent that would be well-regarded by the older adult. Negative face included speech that implied that the speaker did not care about, or had a negative evaluation of, the listener. This speech included criticism, initiating bad news or divisive topics, being uncooperative, marking status, etc. Although positive and polite strategies were often proposed by adult children as a way to initiate conversations with their aging parent about the sensitive issue of eldercare, adult children used negative strategies more frequently in overall conversation (Pitts et al., 2014). Thus, while adult children's proposed initial messages that emphasized love and concern were sensitive to maintaining positive parental "face," other proposed messages showed insensitivity toward aging parents that jeopardized positive "face," including the use of messages that inadvertently communicated ageism (Pitts et al., 2014).

Nevertheless, it is important to point out that older parents may just as easily hold negative stereotypes about the lifestyles and values of younger people they know and hold ageist views about their adult children that could also contribute to communication conflict (Keaton and Giles, 2015). In addition, older people themselves can internalize stereotypes about their own age group, even adjusting their normal behavior to mirror negative age-based behavioral expectations (Christian et al., 2014; Emile et al., 2013; Keaton and Giles, 2015). When negative aged-based stereotypes are played out in communications between adult children and their aging parents, it can result in the reinforcement of such stereotypes—potentially leading to an increase in older adults' anxiety about their own abilities, thereby reducing self-esteem (Begman and Bodner, 2015; Lin and Giles, 2013). Younger generations may see their responsibilities differently and conflict may arise when solutions are presented that go against traditional expectations. Indeed, Tobio (2001) asserts that rapid social or political change increases the differences between generations and limits their communication and the possibility for them to negotiate the complexities of that social change.

Stereotypes that shape parent/adult child communication are not just age-based, but can also be gender-based as well. Because women live longer than men on average, the context of aging itself is highly gendered. Fifty years ago, a person in the United States had about a 50 percent chance of surviving to age 65, but, today, more than two-thirds of women can expect to live until they are at least 80 years old (Mitchell and Bruns, 2010). Thus, predominantly, elderly people in families are women. Older women are the target of stereotypes about both their age and gender. They receive strong contradictory messages, often in the form of jokes and comments, about their aging bodies. The media often portrays older women in terms of their diminished value and uses derogatory language to describe them, and these stereotypes can shape intergenerational family communication (Lin and Giles, 2013).

At the micro, personal level, then, parent/adult child communication can be shaped by negative age- and gender-based stereotypes that can contribute to and shape family conflict.

Social judgment: the bigger picture

The previous section argued that stereotypes about aging and gender can be acquired through over-generalized personal experience and internalized over the course of life. However, it is not only individuals and their internalized age-based stereotypes at the micro level that shape parent/adult child communication, but also age-based stereotypes that are incorporated into policy and practice that may even initiate or exacerbate the parent/adult child communication predicament.

In the larger societal sense, stereotypical myths and generalizations about aging appear to be divided. On the one hand, some people argue that older people use up more than their fair share of healthcare dollars and that they are not only a drain on the "system" but also a burden to families and society (Wiles and Jayasinha, 2013). On the other hand, some people claim that most older adults in Canada are rich and hold accumulated wealth (Office of the Seniors Advocate for British Columbia, 2014). However, facts that are often overlooked in this debate include whether a majority of seniors live independently in their own homes or whether seniors provide financial and grandparental support.

Another societal concern about the aging population is the seemingly greater incidence of neurological disorders and cognitive impairment compared to the past. This concern may stem from the difficulty in differentiating between what are normal age-related changes to body and brain functioning and the changes that are non-normal, such as those associated with Alzheimer's disease (Sachs, 1997). With society's concern about increasing rates of dementia, family members and the individuals affected may misattribute normal behaviors such as confusion and memory loss that can occur due to stress or lack of sleep to non-normal physiological changes that require medical attention and concern. It is also important to point out that the significance of some of the physical and cognitive changes that occur with age is actually socially constructed (American Bar Association,

2010) and the incredible variation among older adults with respect to declines is often overlooked (Salthouse, 2012). In fact, Salthouse (2012) notes that when different people were tested at different ages in different years, it was found that within-cohort differences across ages were as large as between-cohort differences across ages. This provides further support for the argument that social factors can influence cognitive change.

As a psychogeriatric consultant, I saw many families who could provide physical care, but they could not, however, understand or manage the behaviors that often accompany cognitive impairment due to neurological conditions, mental health issues, addictions, medical decline and the effects of medications. Physical changes due to aging can make the older person more fragile and feeble-looking, and neurological changes can affect the person's memory, personality and behaviors. These changes and the responses to them affect the older person's self-image, their role within the family and communication patterns with other family members, including a reluctance to speak up. I find professionally that the family may then focus communication for both parents on the care provider, creating yet another family dynamic. As with all individuals, dignity is enhanced when older parents' opinions are considered and they are able to participate in the decision-making process (Bayer et al., 2005; Sachs, 1997).

Societal concerns about healthcare costs and the growing numbers of older adults needing care have been incorporated into changes to and reductions in government supports and programs for older people. This has resulted in the downloading of many of the responsibilities associated with eldercare from the public to the private/family domain (Killian et al., 2008). The transfer of responsibility for care to the family has particularly been influenced by socially constructed "normative" pressures about filial responsibilities that have been reinforced by the state (Killian et al., 2008).

Szydlik (2008, p. 111) suggests that "state regulations create frameworks in which individuals and families live their private relations." It has often been shown that neoliberal political ideologies encourage the view that older people are an expensive drain on government-provided social services and a burden on younger people, and that "bad" aging is the fault of older people (Douglas, 2014). This negative view of aging may not only affect how service providers regard or treat an older adult's condition (e.g., viewing problems as normal aging instead of as a treatable condition), but it may also affect the older person's view of themselves as a "burden" to society. This attitude has been shown to contribute to problems associated with family communication, particularly at the end of life (Norton et al., 2003).

Thus, stereotypes incorporated into policy can ripple through to shape supports available to aging families and the responsibilities that they need to assume, which, in turn, can initiate family conflict.

Conflict and ambiguity in families

The tension between autonomy and independence has been a topic that has generated much interest among scholars exploring family conflict associated with aging. In general, older adult/adult child relationships are fluid, with fluctuations of interdependence, independence and dependence occurring naturally (Blieszner et al., 1996). Moreover, Blieszner et al. (1996) suggest that when conflict does occur in high-quality relationships, it does not diminish the cohesion between older parents and their adult children.

Intergenerational conflict can occur for a variety of reasons. Offspring may experience stress in the form of filial anxiety, anticipating problems associated with the aging process even when the parent is still healthy and independent (Fingerman, 1996). In addition, the frailty of older parents and their dependence on their children can introduce friction and strain into the intergenerational relationship, especially when adult children struggle with the decision about whether to take over control of financial and/or living arrangements (Sachs, 1997; Silverstein et al., 2010). Control-based conflicts may also emerge when decisions need to be made about driving, or if there is a need for public or private home care support (Sachs, 1997). Moreover, some parents may instigate conflict if they favor one adult child over another as an "investment of moral capital," as not all children within the same family are perceived by parents to be good "bets" as dependable care providers (Silverstein et al., 2012, p. 1259). Conflicting emotions may therefore lead to divisiveness and undermine the support that adult children can or will provide to older parents in need.

Assumptions that support is positive for the recipient and stressful for the provider, however, may not, in reality, be accurate. Conflict may arise if the recipient of care perceives that support to be undermining her/his autonomy. Some family members may also stir up conflict if they deny their older family member's problems to avoid taking responsibility for caregiving tasks, which they may perceive as a frightening burden (Sachs, 1997). Some younger adult children may cause conflict by avoiding older family members; however, some older parents may also consciously cause conflict by avoiding frequent interaction with children, too, in order to maintain their own independence (Smith, 1998). Further studies are needed to determine when support is beneficial or detrimental to both adult children and the older parent (Fingerman et al., 2013).

Research suggests that for aging families, if conflict is combined with emotional cohesion, this can lead to what is called intergenerational ambivalence (Silverstein et al., 2012). The possibility that family members experience an emotional dissonance of simultaneously warm and antagonistic feelings is the basis of Ambivalence Theory (Silverstein et al., 2010). Thus, mixed or contradictory feelings between younger and older family members is an example of intergenerational ambivalence (Lendon et al., 2014).

In Hebblethwaite and Norris' (2010) study of intergenerational ambivalence, grandparents and grandchildren who were interviewed first indicated that they had positive relationships and they struggled to acknowledge contradictory feelings before finally speaking about how they experienced ambivalence. Grandparents felt that they needed to "bite their tongue" or not interfere. Grandchildren did not want to hurt their grandparents' feelings. Ambivalence sometimes resulted from expectations that visits should be positive, when sometimes they were not. In order to overcome negative feelings, grandchildren stated that they focussed on the benefits of learning that they obtained from interacting with their grandparents. The more invested both older and younger family members were in the relationship, the more ambivalence occurred. However, focussing on the perceived benefits of the relationship appeared to make ambivalence more manageable (Hebblethwaite and Norris, 2010).

Birditt et al. (2009) studied constructive, destructive and avoidant strategies that were used to cope with tensions in the parent and grown children's relationships. Constructive strategies predicted relationships with greater quality, while destructive and avoidant strategies predicted greater ambivalence, suggesting that parents and their adult children may benefit from directly confronting problems rather than avoiding them. Both parents and their adult children reported using constructive strategies more often than destructive or avoidant strategies. However, parents reported higher use of constructive strategies. Of interest is that people with more education were found to use more avoidant strategies and that families with fewer resources found more adaptive ways to deal with tensions.

It is also interesting to note that patterns of intergenerational ambivalence remain "fluid and dynamic across the lifespan" (Hebblethwaite and Norris, 2010, p. 503). Yet, Pillemer and Suitor (2002) suggest that ambivalence may be heightened during life course transitions, for either adult children or older adults. For example, their data show a strong relationship between interpersonal stress and ambivalence, suggesting that the presence of ambivalence may also be a good predictor of parents' well-being.

Silverstein et al. (2010) acknowledge that the simultaneous presence of affection and conflict in intergenerational relationships is obvious to anyone who is part of a family. However, for researchers it can be a challenging concept to measure. Furthermore, Fingerman et al. (2013) suggest that Intergenerational Ambivalence Theory may not adequately acknowledge the complexity of the parent–child relationship. Additional research is needed to fill this gap.

Conclusion and suggestions for practice

The changing diversity of family structures and mobility patterns, as well as changing government policies, have all shaped intergenerational communication in the modern era. Internalized stereotypes that are generated at both the micro and societal levels have contributed to a communication predicament between aging parents and their adult children. In the interpersonal micro sense, ageist stereotypes are internalized early in life. Age-based stereotypes that are then integrated into communication reinforce myths about aging and affect the self-confidence and agency of older adults. Societal concerns about aging and government healthcare spending conflict with contrasting concerns about wealthy seniors. Internalized stereotypes about aging and gender that are incorporated into political ideologies, policies and services put unfair challenges on families and affect parent/adult child communication.

When conflict is combined with emotional cohesion between generations, it can lead to intergenerational ambivalence. However, researchers suggest that further studies on this theoretical approach need to better tease out the complexity inherent in the parent/adult child relationship.

Recommendations from scholars, social workers, service providers and policy analysts to assist parents and adult children in communicating about issues associated with eldercare are diverse. However, some suggestions follow common themes. For example, building more positive opportunities for intergenerational communication and experiences in our society in general is suggested by Lin and Giles (2013) as an important starting point. Because caregiving is an intimate and intense intergenerational exchange, conflicts between parents and adult children can emerge and may escalate into abuse. A communicative approach provides ways in which abuse can be revealed, interventions identified or problems avoided (Lin and Giles, 2013). Public awareness campaigns such as those recently aired on Canadian television about elder abuse may help people to think about age- or gender-related stereotypes, abuse of power and the impact that this has on others (see: www.youtube.com/watch?v=OP0sZB9jRlA).

Kramer et al. (2010) suggest that when service providers and social workers are making assessments, they need to involve multiple family members and to obtain a careful history of family functioning and relationship quality. This may help to identify families at risk of conflict. In particular, professionals need to pay attention to unresolved conflicts and the varying perceptions of a parent's health status among family members. They also suggest that family meetings may assist in building trust between practitioners, adult children and parents and in facilitating an exchange of information across generations, thereby enhancing communication

Mitchell and Bruns (2010) assert that by engaging older women in reflection about how they understand themselves in relation to others, and why some things are perceived by others to be outside of an older adult's control, is essential to this work. Deconstructing assumptions associated with responsibility and "natural" talents is important in dispelling myths that are often internalized and acted out in communication. The stereotype associated with age and decline in physical functioning is often viewed as a sign of weakness, leaving women feeling ashamed and embarrassed about their bodies (Mitchell and Bruns, 2010). Mitchell and Bruns (2010) suggest that it is important to change the media narrative about aging and to teach clients the skills to question messages about health, beauty and the aging body. Edwards and Chapman (2004) highlight the Model for Health Promoting Communication as an intervention that can assist in clarifying role expectations. They suggest that this model can facilitate the negotiation of roles not only within the family, but also for health professionals working with families, thus raising awareness of stereotypical role expectations and their outcomes in parent/adult child communication.

An understanding of the communication predicament between adult children and their aging parents is contextual, complex and fluid. It is clear that the messages from the 1990s still resonate today.

References

American Bar Association. (2010). *Assessment of Older Adults with Diminished Capacity: A Handbook for Psychologists*. Chicago, IL: American Bar Association.

Bayer, T., Tadd, W. and Krajcik, S. (2005). Dignity: The voice of older people. *Quality in Ageing*, 6(1), 22–29.

Begman, Y.S. and Bodner, E. (2015). Ageist attitudes block young adults' ability for compassion toward incapacitated older adults. *International Psychogeriatrics*, 27(9), 1541–1550.

Birditt, K.S., Rott, L.M. and Fingerman, K.L. (2009). "If you can't say something nice, don't say anything at all": Coping with interpersonal tensions in the parent–child relationship during adulthood. *Journal of Family Psychology*, 23(6), 769–778.

Birditt, K.S., Miller, L.M., Fingerman, K.L. and Lefkowitz, E.S. (2009). Tensions in the parent and adult child relationship: Links to solidarity and ambivalence. *Psychology and Aging*, 24(2), 287–295.

Blieszner, R., Usita, P.M. and Mancini, J.A. (1996). Diversity and dynamics in late-life mother–daughter relationships. *Journal of Women & Aging*, 8(3–4), 5–24.

Bodner, E., Bergman, Y.S. and Cohen Fridel, S. (2012). Different dimensions of ageist attitudes among men and women: A multigenerational perspective. *International Psychogeriatrics*, 24(6), 895–901.

Christian, J., Turner, R., Holt, N., Larkin, M. and Cotler, J.H. (2014). Does intergenerational contact reduce ageism? When and how contact interventions actually work? *Journal of Arts and Humanities*, 3(1), 1–15.

Cruikshank, M. (2013). *Learning to be Old: Gender, Culture and Aging* (3rd ed). Lanham, MD: Rowman & Littlefield.

Douglas, S. (2014). Still living with sexism (after all these years). *Soundings: A Journal of Politics and Culture*, 58(Winter 2014–15), 34–43.

Edwards, H. and Chapman, H. (2004). Caregiver–care receiver communication part 2: Overcoming the influence of stereotypical role expectations. *Quality in Aging*, 5(3), 3–12.

Emile, M., Chalabaev, A., Stephan, Y., Corrion, K. and d'Arripe-Longueville, F. (2013). Aging stereotypes and active lifestyle: Personal correlates of stereotype internalization and relationships with level of physical activity among older adults. *Psychology of Sport & Exercise*, 15, 198–204.

Fingerman, K.L. (1996). Sources of tension in the aging mother and adult daughter relationship. *Psychology and Aging*, 11(4), 591–606.

Fingerman, K., Sechrist, J. and Birditt, K. (2013). Changing views on intergenerational ties. *Gerontology*, 59(1), 64–70.

Harwood, J., Rittenour, C.E. and Lin, M. (2013). Family communications in later life. In A.L. Vangelisti (ed.), *The Routledge Handbook of Family Communication* (pp. 112–126). New York: Routledge.

Hebblethwaite, S. and Norris, J.E. (2010). "You don't want to hurt his feelings...": Family leisure as a context for intergenerational ambivalence. *Journal of Leisure Research*, 42(3), 489–508.

Hummert, M.L., Garstka, T.A., Shaner, J.L. and Strahm, S. (1994). Stereotypes of the elderly held by young, middle-aged, and elderly adults. *Journals of Gerontology, Series B: Psychological Sciences and Social Sciences*, 49(5), 240–249.

Keaton, S.A. and Giles, H. (2015). Subjective health: The roles of communication, language, aging, stereotypes and culture. *International Journal of Society, Culture & Language*, (In Press).

Killian, C., Salmoni, A., Ward-Griffin, C. and Kloseck, M. (2008). Perceiving falls within a family context: A focused ethnographic approach. *Canadian Journal on Aging*, 27(4), 331–345.

Kramer, B.J., Kavanaugh, M., Trentham-Dietz, A., Walsh, M. and Yonker, J.A. (2010). Predictors of family conflict at the end of life: The experiences of spouses and adult children of persons living with lung cancer. *The Gerontologist*, 50(2), 215–225.

Lendon, J.P., Silverstein, M. and Giarrusso, R. (2014). Ambivalence in older parent–adult child relationships: Mixed feelings, mixed measures. *Journal of Marriage and Family*, 76(2), 272–284.

Levy, B. (2009). Stereotype embodiment: A psychosocial approach to aging. *Current Directions in Psychological Science*, 18(6), 332–336.

Lin, M.C. and Giles, H. (2013). The dark side of family communication: A communication model of elder abuse and neglect. *International Psychogeriatrics*, 25(8), 1275–1280.

Mitchell, V. and Bruns, C.M. (2010). Writing one's own story: Women, aging and the social narrative. *Women & Therapy*, 34(1–2), 114–128.

Norton, S.A., Tilden, V.P., Tolle, S.W., Nelson, C.A. and Talamantes Eggman, S. (2003). Life support withdrawal: Communication and conflict. *American Journal of Critical Care*, 12(6), 548–555.

Office of the Seniors Advocate for British Columbia. (2014). Stereotyping seniors as wealthy not reality for many seniors. Retrieved from www.seniorsadvocatebc.ca/osa-reports/stereotyping-seniors-as-wealthy-not-reality-for-many-seniors.

Ontario Human Rights Commision. (n.d.). *The Changing Face of Canadian Families*. Toronto, ON: OHRC, Retrieved from www.ohrc.on.ca/en/human-rights-and-family-ontario/changing-face-canadian-families.

Pillemer, K. and Suitor, J.J. (2002). Explaining mothers' ambivalence toward their adult children. *Journal of Marriage and Family*, 64(3), 602–613.

Pitts, M.J., Fowler, C., Fisher, C.L. and Smith, S.A. (2014). Politeness stategies in imagined conversation openers about eldercare. *Journal of Language and Social Psychology*, 33(1), 29–48.

Powell, V. (1996). Is there a communication predicament between adult children and their aging parents? In G. Joseph (ed.), *Difficult Issues in Aging in Difficult Times*. Guelph, ON: University of Guelph.

Ryan, E.B., Giles, H., Bartolucci, G. and Henwood, K. (1986). Psycholinguistic and social psychological components of communication by and with the elderly. *Language and Communication*, 6(1/2), 1–24.

Ryan, E.B., Hummert, M.L. and Boich, L.H. (1995). Communication predicaments of aging: Patronizing behaviour toward older adults. *Journal of Language and Social Psychology*, 14(1/2), 144–166.

Sachs, P.R. (1997). Short-term treatment for families of older adults with neurological impairments. *American Journal of Family Therapy*, 25(4), 345–356.

Salthouse, T. (2012). Consequences of age-related cognitive declines. *Annual Review of Psychology*, 63, 201–226.

Silverstein, M., Conroy, S.J. and Gans, D. (2012). Beyond solidarity, reciprocity and altruism: Moral capital as a unifying concept in intergenerational support for older people. *Ageing & Society*, 32(7), 1246–1262.

Silverstein, M., Gans, D., Lowenstein, A., Giarrusso, R. and Bengtson, V.L. (2010). Older parent–child relationships in six developed nations: Comparisons at the intersection of affection and conflict. *Journal of Marriage and Family*, 72(4), 805–1038.

Smith, G.C. (1998). Geographic separation and patterns of social interaction between residents of senior citizen apartment buildings and their adult children. *The Canadian Geographer*, 42(2), 145–158.

Szydlik, M. (2008). Intergenerational solidarity and conflict. *Journal of Comparative Family Studies*, 39(1), 97–114.

Tobio, C. (2001). Working and mothering: Women's strategies in Spain. *European Societies*, 3(3), 339–371.

Wiles, J.L. and Jayasinha, R. (2013). Care for place: The contributions older people make to their communities. *Journal of Aging Studies*, 27, 93–101.

Williams, A. and Nussbaum, J.F. (2001). *Intergenerational Communication Across the Life Span*. New York: Digital Printing by Routledge.

8 Neoliberalism, temporary foreign workers and precarious eldercare/eldercare work

Gillian Joseph and Belinda Leach

In 1996, Gillian Joseph wrote about how Canadian free trade agreements were reshaping eldercare policy (Joseph, 1996). Twenty years later, free trade is one plank in a far broader set of practices and ideologies commonly referred to as neoliberalism. This chapter asks how the elements of neoliberalism converge to shape current conditions for eldercare in Canada. State social supports have been reduced, or are available only privately at a cost and through markets that exist in some but not all regions of the country, in step with neoliberal ideas that download responsibility for care to the individual and her or his family. It has been noted that the impacts of such cutbacks have been felt most acutely by women as both recipients and providers of care. Indeed, Federici (2012) argues that the provision of eldercare is essentially a gender issue—addressed increasingly through the services of documented and undocumented migrant women care workers as a cost-effective solution for families and institutions. In Canada, foreign care workers are recruited through the longstanding Live-in Caregiver Program (LCP) designed originally to bring migrant women into the country to perform childcare, but recently modified to address the growing need for eldercare.

We view neoliberalism as a political and ideological framework that has two particular consequences for the investigation of eldercare as both need and service. First, under neoliberalism the state withdraws from certain regulatory and service provision roles, giving rise to precarity in both care need and care work. Second, under neoliberalism, the state intervenes in very specific ways to reshape immigration policy, leading to growing numbers of temporary migrant care workers with precarious citizenship and work status. We argue that while temporary migrant worker programs may promise a tempting option for both care recipients and care providers, they fail to address the needs and realities of the people involved. Using a feminist intersectionality approach, we review aspects of, and debates about, these policy shifts to argue that the conjuncture of political trends and the lived realities of women result in an environment of eldercare in Canada that can be characterized as precarious work and precarious care.

Neoliberalism and precarious care work

Ganti (2014) identifies the principles of neoliberalism as the deregulation of the economy, including liberalization of trade and privatization, new roles for labour, capital and the state, market exchange as guiding human action, and a self-regulating free market ruled by competition and self-interest. In fact, it is disturbing to note that the tenets of neoliberalism are so internalized that for many people they now constitute an unquestioned "common-sense" understanding of the modern world.

Neoliberalism was introduced onto the world stage via economic reforms in Latin America in the 1950s and 1960s. These, and subsequently other developing economies, were radically restructured and transformed, giving rise to political, social and economic crises fueled by the "tremendous social inequality" that resulted (Ganti, 2014, p. 93). Two elements of this social inequality are especially relevant to our analysis. First, people in the global south sought routes to higher wage countries through migration. Second, precarity emerged as a broad social condition for many people globally, but especially in work. Scholars have suggested that *neoliberalism* and *precarity* are deeply intertwined and inseparable, the latter being the outcome of the former (Burrows, 2013; Standing, 2011). The study of eldercare requires an understanding of their influence in shaping the experience of both providing and receiving care.

Precarious work has increased in Canada and elsewhere since the 1970s (Kalleberg, 2013), particularly affecting workers in the healthcare sector (Armstrong and Armstrong, 2009). The Law Commission of Ontario (2010) defines precarious work as short term with few benefits and little security or control, factors that contribute to worker vulnerability and a related decline in full-time and secure employment with a liveable wage. The detrimental effects of this shift have been felt in many aspects of people's lives. Migrant care workers were singled out by the Law Commission as a group in Canada who are especially vulnerable because of the precarious nature of their work and lives, an issue of increasing concern around the world. In these terms, care work exemplifies precarious work.

While we highlight the precarious nature of care *work* under neoliberalism, it is equally important to recognize the precarious nature of care *provision* from the perspectives of the recipients. Reductions in social supports for the elderly are a consequence of neoliberal doctrine globally (Federici, 2012). Combined with ill-defined or absent rights of care workers, the care relationship becomes more precarious for providers and recipients, because neither can depend on a stable care process (Armstrong and Armstrong, 2009). Inconsistent access to services for the elderly across Canada, together with declining programs and supports and a lack of standardized care, renders all eldercare precarious (Verbeeten et al., 2015). In private home care, concerns about qualifications, lengthy and costly processing, third party employee management and the absence of adequate government monitoring systems threaten health, safety, economic security and consistency of care (Marchitelli, 2015; Migneault, 2015). Proponents of neoliberalism assert that patients are now "customers" who can choose how they are cared for, but they forget that elderly people engage with the healthcare system not as a luxury, but because their aging bodies require it. Under these circumstances there is no choice; the recipient of care is in a very precarious position indeed.

Neoliberal thinking has also reshaped immigration policy. In Canada, the programs in place since the 1960s to bring in permanent residents (about 250,000 per year for the past decade) have now been overtaken by temporary foreign worker (TFW) programs that bring in twice as many people each year. These programs are closely tied to regional and temporal shifts in labour market needs, with the claim that they are flexible and responsive to employer needs and labour market gaps. For their critics, however, TFW programs produce a category of migrant denied fundamental rights of citizenship, including rights to employment mobility (Hennebry and Preibisch, 2012). As numerous critics have pointed out, workers who come to Canada under these conditions have precarious status, neither fully protected by law nor offering stability of income, making them vulnerable to exploitation by employers (Bakan and Stasiulis, 2005; Giles and Arat-Koc, 1994).

TFW programs have expanded globally and clearly encompass principles of neoliberalism. The longstanding Live-in Caregiver Program (LCP), which we describe in more detail below, is one form of TFW program. In 2013, LCP workers represented 15 percent of all TFWs in Canada (Migrant Mothers Project, 2015). As a product of an earlier phase of pre-neoliberal immigration policy (Leach, 2013), the LCP deviates from neoliberal principles in certain ways. Most importantly, it permits a pathway to citizenship that is absent in other "low-skill" TFW programs. It is important to recognize, however, that it remains at root a *temporary* worker program with considerably more hurdles for acquiring permanent residency than permanent programs.

Precarious care, then, references both *care workers* subject to particular kinds of immigration policies and *care recipients* subject to the reduced provision and monitoring of care from the state. For both, their lives are shaped by dependency, lack of information, instability, vulnerability and danger.

An intersectional approach to precarious eldercare

We view the nexus of neoliberalism, migrant care workers and precarious eldercare work through the lens of intersectionality. This approach suggests that race and gender should not be considered as independent identities, but as overlapping or intersecting interactions of gender, sexuality, class, age and race that must be viewed in relation to systems of oppression, power and discrimination (Crenshaw, 1989). Intersectionality theory has been particularly important in feminist scholarship (Few-Demo, 2014; Mahler et al., 2015). The power of the approach is in its ability to capture experiences of discrimination that arise from the intersection of multiple grounds. Intersectionality is particularly useful for examining how people are differently positioned socially and vis-à-vis the state, to show how neoliberalism reinforces racial and gendered hierarchies and "redefines the terms of citizenship" (Fisher, 2006, p. 55).

Our engagement with intersectionality follows Greenwood (2008) who identifies its key assumptions, each with implications for our study of eldercare. For example, the complexity of social identities may cause conflict within an individual, such as a feminist who believes in women's power and autonomy but acts out of fear for the safety of an elderly parent. Social identities are grounded in both ideology and symbolism, rendering women with grey hair and wrinkles as invisible and powerless (Calasanti and King, 2015), with serious implications for the valuing of eldercare and eldercare work and of elderly women's agency. Social identities are also historically and contextually situated. For example, historically, women in families were considered responsible for providing eldercare. As more women enter the workforce and as rural-to-urban migration of youth increases, this expectation becomes problematic (Joseph et al., 2007; Lero and Joseph, 2007). Finally, identities operate within and are shaped by structures of power. Thus, for some older women, being poor in old age is linked to pension policies that ignore the unstable nature of women's careers due to the demands of child and eldercare (Benefits Canada, 2015; Ontario Human Rights Commission, 2000).

Despite its relevance to the study of aging, feminist intersectionality theory has not been used extensively in gerontology (Calasanti and King, 2015). In fact, studies on aging and older women have been scarce in feminist research, possibly reflecting a cultural gerontophobia (Freixas et al., 2012). This continuing oversight perpetuates the invisibility of older women and ignores the relationships of power that shape not only the experiences of older women and men themselves, but also the experiences of and attitudes about those who care for them by association (Federici, 2012; Schwiter et al., 2015). This, in turn, shapes the policies and practices that affect older women in need and their caregivers. The failure to link these areas of scholarship means that few studies have applied intersectionality to migrant care work. This is particularly troubling since people's lives frequently span national borders through which they encounter social, political and ideological forces increasingly associated with globalized policies and practices (Few-Demo, 2014).

So we tilt the theoretical lens of intersectionality in two directions: first, to explore how neoliberal principles shape the gendered responsibility for eldercare itself, creating the demand for foreign care workers, and in the other direction to consider how neoliberal policies and practices shape the experience of being a migrant eldercare worker.

State restructuring and gendered caregiving

The offloading of responsibility for eldercare to individuals and families has been an important outcome of neoliberal-inspired change. This offloading has had a significant impact on both informal and formal sectors of care work globally (Federici, 2012). As a result, the demand for care workers around the globe has intensified, for both home- and institutional-based care settings (Lee and Johnstone, 2013) and this gendered phenomenon has become "one of the most pressing issues of our times" (Chatterjee, 2011, p. 456).

Historically, responsibility for unpaid caregiving fell to women in families (Cangiano, 2014; Federici, 2012). In recent decades, women have been less available to meet the increasing need for unpaid eldercare as a result of population aging, declining birthrates, changing family roles, precarious work schedules, migration patterns, changing perspectives on responsibility for care and cuts in government services (Keefe, 2011). For families who cannot afford private substitute care, it is women who tend to reduce their employment to provide unpaid care for elderly family members, sacrificing their earnings and pensions and creating a paradox whereby the more women care for others, the less care they will receive themselves in old age (Federici, 2012).

For wealthier families experiencing these pressures, and within institutionalized care settings too, there is growing reliance on documented and undocumented migrant caregivers (Cangiano, 2014; Federici, 2012). The movement of migrant labour from south to north (and from south to south) to meet this need has led to "global care chains" where a family care worker in one country is replaced by someone else from outside of the family and from a poorer country. In turn, the migrant worker is replaced as care provider in her own family by someone else (Federici, 2012; Lee and Johnstone, 2013). Migrant workers who move from poorer countries to wealthier, healthier countries often leave behind significant challenges for their own family caregivers, including burdens of disease and disability, rapidly growing elderly populations, and fewer resources and supports (Eckenwiler, 2014; Faraday, 2014).

In North America and Europe, eldercare is a low-skilled, marginalized sector of employment, characterized by precariousness, with low pay, poor working conditions and high turnover (Armstrong, 2009; Cangiano, 2014). One aspect of this marginalization relates to the location of the work, in a private home. This transforms personal space into both public *and* private space, containing formal *and* informal work, and dependent *and* independent identities (Schwiter et al., 2015). Because the home as workplace is shielded from public scrutiny, it keeps workers and their situations isolated, invisible and thereby vulnerable to abuse (Schwiter et al., 2015; Urbano, 2011).

Traditionally considered to be "women's work," care work has been devalued and this has made it very difficult to attract local paid workers (Roberts, 2014). The absence of a comprehensive eldercare policy in many countries, including Canada, has perpetuated a marginalized care system and contributed to a reliance on low-cost migrant care workers (Eckenwiler,

2014). A lack of planning for an aging health workforce has also exacerbated recruitment and retention problems locally, in turn contributing to the downloading of responsibility for care to families as health workers retire and are not replaced (Joseph et al., 2007). Consequently, women in female-dominated professions such as nursing and home healthcare work have become an integral part of the global economy in one of the fastest growing sectors of migrant employment (Eckenwiler, 2014).

Not only is it predominantly women who take up paid and unpaid care work, but because of life expectancy patterns that favour women, older women are more likely to be recipients of care in later life (Lero and Joseph, 2007). Thus, the feminization of care work and of the aged population itself has made elderly people and their caregivers a low political priority, seemingly of little importance, with inadequate policies and services (Federici, 2012). This political marginalization is particularly critical. Canada has refused to recognize those who provide front-line, hands-on care to elderly people in nursing homes and public-funded homecare as regulated healthcare professionals (CBC News, 2010). Moreover, eldercare provided institutionally and in the community is not deemed an essential service under the Canada Health Care Act because it is not viewed as "medically necessary"; something that has been drawn to the attention of government policy makers for some time (Romanow, 2002, p. 63).

Migrant care work: then and now

Migrant caregiving in Canada has historically been subject to political forces, and this has resulted in precarious outcomes for migrants. It is now increasingly shaped by the neoliberal principles that underlie immigration policy. The possible pathways for migrants to reach a host country carry expectations and practices associated with gender, class, race and age, as well as other identities (Leach, 2013). In the Canadian context, the two longstanding TFW programs produce gendered migration streams—seasonal agricultural work for men and live-in caregiving work for women.

By 1955, Canada had agreements with Jamaica and Barbados whereby single women were admitted as landed immigrants as long as they remained in live-in service for one year (Brickner and Straehle, 2010). This was the beginning of a link between gendered domestic work and access to permanent residency. In the early 1970s, access to permanent residency was withdrawn, and there was public outcry at reports of exploitation and abuse of workers, issues that continue to plague migrant care workers today.

By 1981, the program returned to allow access to landed immigrant status at the end of a three-year work period (Brickner and Straehle, 2010). It also allowed domestic workers to apply to bring their children, consistent with the principle of family reunification. The program was intended to fill the growing need for staff in daycare centres, thus serving the needs of parents and children, but not addressing broader care needs. In 1991, the LCP was established, also addressing the childcare gap. Citizenship and Immigration Canada data show the number of caregivers with a valid work permit to have grown from 15,000 in 2004 to over 32,000 in 2008, declining to 16,000 in 2013 (Migrant Mothers Project, 2015). Despite its designation as a low-skill occupation, not requiring high levels of formal education, applicants are increasingly well-educated (Kelly et al., 2011) and they are also required to seek specific training before coming to Canada (Gardiner Barber and Bryan, 2012). Indeed, Bourgeault et al. (2010) found that over 44 percent of migrant care workers were working as nurses prior to migrating to Canada.

In 2014, the program was revised in response to growing concerns and lobbying efforts about abuse due to the nature of the employee/employer contractual relationship and workers' live-in arrangements. The live-in requirement was eliminated (though it remains an option), and the program was renamed the Caregiver Program. The revised program also created two "pathways": one for caregivers of children and the other for caregivers of people with high medical needs.

Those seeking a caregiver under the program must first obtain a Labour Market Impact Assessment (LMIA) to ensure that no Canadian worker is available. Faraday (2014) notes that most employers use a third party agency to recruit, that some agencies have been accused of exploiting workers, and that workers who complain have sometimes found themselves or their communities punished by being cut out of the recruitment process. Once the LMIA is granted and a caregiver hired, a contract is drawn up and the caregiver must apply for a Canadian work permit. The employee then receives a temporary resident visa and can begin work. The employer is required to complete the record of employment for the employee and, after at least 24 months of work, she can apply for permanent residency status. If the employee is terminated, she may be qualified to apply for employment insurance until a new employer has acquired a new LMIA (Government of Canada, 2015).

However, there have been significant snags in the revised policy. Caregivers wanting to improve their status as qualified healthcare professionals in order to earn higher wages have argued that they cannot get professional licences from accredited bodies without a work permit, but they cannot get a work permit until they have a Canadian license (Salami et al., 2014; Tungohan, 2015). There have also been lengthy delays in processing new applications as well as delays processing applications for residency from caregivers who have fulfilled the employment requirements (Boudreau, 2015). Caregiver organizations also noted a troubling trend in early 2015, with extremely low numbers of approvals of LMIAs in the childcare stream (two of 169 in January, 16 of 262 in March). Interestingly, in the high medical needs stream, approval rates were higher (12 of 26 in January, 27 of 35 in March) (Association of Caregiver and Nanny Agencies Canada, 2015). Nevertheless, the Caregiver Program remains the only TFW program that can result in permanent residency status and family reunification for low-skilled temporary workers in Canada (Brickner and Straehle, 2010).

Caregivers and global inequality

As the Caregiver Program has evolved and TFW programs have expanded, source countries for care workers have changed too. The Philippines has become the top source country for Canadian immigrants, with Filipinos representing the majority of participants in the Caregiver Program and a major source country for private caregivers globally (Faraday, 2014). In 2006, of the more than 8.5 million Filipinos working abroad, domestic workers comprised 29.7 percent (Urbano, 2011). Filipino domestic workers can be found from Singapore to Oman and in Europe, the United States and Australia (Urbano, 2011). More than 40,000 Filipinos became Canadian permanent residents in 2014 (Canadian Immigration News, 2015).

The global diaspora of migrant care workers from the Philippines has been shaped by histories of colonialism and imperialism that left a legacy of inequality and poverty (Urbano, 2011). More recently, it has also been shaped by the pressures of neoliberal restructuring inflicted by international financial institutions such as the International Monetary Fund (Eckenwiler, 2014). The commodification of Filipino migrant care workers began in the 1970s as a temporary fix for rising unemployment rates in the Philippines and a balance of payments/international debt crisis after the 1980s (Guerrero, 2000). Although it is not the poorest socio-economic group that leaves, since costs associated with passports, visas, etc. can be high, many migrants move because they lack employment opportunities and have poor living conditions (Faraday, 2014). This situation is exacerbated by foreign investment trade flows, world market prices, interest rates and military activity, all associated with neoliberal policies that force countries to liberalize their economic systems (Urbano, 2011). Countries such as the Philippines were pressured to increase taxes and reduce spending on social supports to avoid defaulting on debt payments, creating significant hardship (Gundzik, 2005). The World Trade Organization also contributes to this struggle by imposing high duties and tariffs on export products and reducing agricultural subsidies, among other measures (Urbano, 2011).

In response to these conditions, the Philippines government set up education and recruitment agencies to train nurses and other care workers so they could find employment in higher-income countries (Gardiner Barber and Bryan, 2012). Remittances from these migrants have become important to the nation's economy (Lee and Johnstone, 2013). In Manila, close to half the total population is directly dependent on this income (Faraday, 2014). Overseas employment is no longer a short-term solution in the Philippines but rather an ongoing feature of the government's development plan (Urbano, 2011). This underscores the importance of migrant workers for the economic survival of Filipino families and for their nation as a whole. Yet despite these broad benefits, migrant workers commonly complain about exploitation and abuse.

The Philippines government has created a comprehensive legal and institutional framework to help migrants with the migration process, including assistance when they return home (Salvador, 2015). Mandatory health coverage, insurance and family assistance programs also provide an important safety net. In Canada, however, concern about protecting migrant workers has not been a priority. Although both the United States and Canada have expressed concerns about the vulnerability of migrant labourers, neither were among the 38 countries that signed the United Nations International Convention on the Protection of the Rights of All Migrant Workers and Members of their Families (Urbano, 2011). One of the reasons the Conservative government of the time gave for not signing was that "signing and ratifying the Convention would force Canada to review its temporary migrants programs in order to make them more respectful of the Convention" (Piche et al., 2006, p. 3). Clearly, the Philippines remains vulnerable to stronger global powers, which in turn contributes to its continuing cycle of poverty.

Precarious work and precarious care: highlighting the intersections

The power of neoliberalism to control and shape the experience of caregivers and care recipients through policy and practice provides a rich tapestry of intersecting threads worthy of careful examination. Issues of power and control can be teased out from the standpoint of the family in need of care or the migrant worker hired to provide that care, highlighting people's specific experiences in their personal worlds of family and work as well as in relation to broader structures and changes in society. When applied to eldercare, neoliberalism defines the issue through a market-based framework of demand and supply, suggesting that care relationships can be viewed as "rational" economic contracts and ignoring many aspects of what it is to be human (Barker, 2012). Neoliberalism defines the elderly person and her/his family as a *consumer* and downloads to them the responsibility for meeting their own needs, independent of government assistance, through private participation in the market (Verbeeten et al., 2015). Similarly, neoliberalism defines the care worker as a *commodity* that can be used, traded and discarded (Hoppania and Vaittinen, 2014).

Taking *unpaid* family eldercare as a starting point for exploring multiple identities, we can see how those associated with gender, age, class and ability come together in eldercare, moulded by neoliberal ideology and practice. Gender is a critical factor in the neoliberal restructuring that offloads responsibilities for eldercare to families, and predominantly to the women in them, in the absence of state-sponsored community services or supports.

The impact of demography, declining services and a lack of a national elder-care strategy is even more significant with respect to gender as it intersects with age, given that women are not only the primary providers of care, but also the primary recipients of care in old age. Neoliberalism perpetuates age-ism and the marginalization of older adults by promoting a stereotypical view of them as fragile, infirm and cognitively inadequate. This ageism and its impact is reflected in the reform of the Caregiver Program through the crea-tion of two new care work *pathways,* one for work with children and the other combining work with the elderly with work for people with disabili-ties and chronic diseases. Ignoring the distinction between developmental changes associated with aging and acute or progressive disability permits a form of ageism and ableism in which aging is defined as illness. This view of aging in neoliberal policy underlies cuts to preventative initiatives such as eye and hearing exams, and is often justified by inferences that older adults are a drain on social services (Sher, 2015). Class intersects with gender and age in two ways: first, as the market expands to fill the gaps from declining services, but only for those who can purchase services, and second, as the market for caregiver labour renders it low value, producing low incomes for those who work there.

Taking *paid* eldercare—such as provided by migrant workers through the Caregiver Program—as a second starting point for exploring multi-ple identities, we can see how gender, race, religion and culture combine, shaped by the power of neoliberalism. Because women are seen as natural caregivers and because they can be paid lower wages compared to men, migrant women are sought to fill the role of eldercare providers. In Canada, women caregivers may immigrate autonomously but they must arrive with-out dependents. Research suggests that many social problems occur when migrant workers leave their families in the care of others. This includes impacts on the psychological health and educational attainment of children and the physical health of older family caregivers, which in turn causes psy-chological stress for the caregiver in Canada (Guerrero, 2000). Within the caregiver program, gender fuels opportunities for exploitation, and physical and psychological abuse, particularly when women are seen as the embodi-ment of a commodity purchased rather than as a person with rights and needs (Guerrero, 2000).

Neoliberalism also shapes caregivers' experience as gender intersects with religion and culture (Tibe Bonifacio and Angeles, 2010). Caring for family is important in Filipino culture and elderly people are highly respected. In contrast to neoliberal ideology that emphasizes individualism, Filipino cul-ture draws on families, regional affiliations and peer groups for support (de Torres, 2002) and this view shapes Filipino caregivers' practices in Canada. Since services for migrants are often inadequate in Canada (Tibe Bonifacio and Angeles, 2010), migrant caregivers turn to community-based organiza-tions such as churches for support and to gain a sense of community (Creese, 2011; Tibe Bonifacio and Angeles, 2010). However, also at the intersection of gender and culture, Filipino women are essentialized as care workers and encouraged to migrate because they stereotypically match Canadian neoliberal ideas of "good citizens" who are self-sufficient, hardworking and efficient (Root et al., 2014), putting them at greater risk for exploitation and abuse (Root et al., 2014; Valbuena, 2013).

Concluding thoughts on migrant eldercare work in the contemporary period

The newly revised Caregiver Program clearly addresses some of the short-comings of the older variants. The option of living outside the employer's home has been demanded by advocates for decades and faster application processing times are intended to enhance family reunification. On the other hand, because care workers must now lock into either working for children or working for those with high medical needs, it has become more difficult for them to accumulate the 24 months they need for permanent residency. Recent changes do not fundamentally change the exploitive elements of the program. As long as workers remain tied to a single employer, they are vulnerable to abuse and exploitation. The live-out option fails to address the roots of this vulnerability. Employers can demand that caregivers live in their homes, making alternatives risky, and without a living wage most are unable to afford to live out anyway—so there is no real choice. Similarly, the promise to process applications quickly for permanent residency will have limited benefits, given the reality of medical and security screening to apply for permanent residency status.

Temporary foreign worker policies make care work and care work-ers invisible, leaving both worker and recipient, and the contractual and social relationship between them, hidden in private spaces. Similarly the details—of applying for permanent residence, seeking appropriate training and credentials, applying for permanent work and reuniting families—are both daunting and obscured. Not only do caregivers face onerous employment conditions and hurdles to permanency, transitioning into the Canadian labour market may be difficult because their work trajectory has been shaped by having to take costly educational upgrading courses while working in "survival" jobs and serving as their families' sole breadwinner. Instead of addressing systemic issues, blame for the program's shortcom-ings shifts to the worker, who with little formal protection is vulnerable to reprisals from her employer.

The provision of eldercare through migrant women's labour is an excel-lent example of the intersectionality of multiple identities, carrying with them associated forms of discrimination and oppression. This process is facilitated through de-regulation and free trade agreements (Roberts and Mahtani, 2010). Eldercare work is feminized—low status, low pay and invisible. Women are discounted and devalued and positioned as subordi-nate. The separation of public and private spheres, deeply evident in migrant care work, degrades the important social role of caring and overburdens women. As Lister (2007) argues, and as our analysis shows, care is deeply political in that it links private spaces with the public and with the global.

Recent political promises from a new Canadian government pledge changes to immigration policy that could bring improvements particularly relevant to eldercare. For example, the Liberal government has stated its plan to eliminate the $1,000 LMIA fee for the care of family members with physical or mental challenges, benefitting those already struggling with the high costs associated with family eldercare (Dery, 2015). It remains to be seen if these changes will meet their objectives. In the words of Pearl S. Buck (1954, p. 337), "the test of a civilization is the way that it cares for its helpless members."

References

Armstrong, P. (2009, May 1). Long-term care problems. *The Monitor*. Retreived from www.policyalternatives.ca/publications/monitor/long-term-care-problems.

Armstrong, P. and Armstrong, H. (2009). Precarious employment in the healthcare sector. In L.F. Vosko, M. MacDonald and I. Campbell (eds), *Gender and the Contours of Precarious Employment*, New York: Routledge.

Association of Caregiver and Nanny Agencies Canada. (2015). *April 2015 Stats Show Only Limited Positive LMIAs Approvals for Caregivers*. Retrieved from www.acnacanada.ca/acna-news/april-2015-lmia-stats-show-more-bleak-numbers-for-approvals.

Bakan, A. and Stasiulis, D. (2005). *Negotiating Citizenship: Migrant Women in Canada and the Global System*. Toronto: University of Toronto Press.

Barker, D.K. (2012). Querying the paradox of caring labor. *Rethinking Marxism*, 4(October), 574–591.

Benefits Canada (2015, September 9). *Women Face Gender Pension Gap*. Retrieved from www.benefitscanada.com/news/women-face-gender-pension-gap-71397.

Boudreau, E. (2015, September, 2). Caregivers' situation worsens under new rules. *Catholic Register*. Retrieved from www.catholicregister.org/item/20803-caregivers-situation-worsens-under-new-rules.

Bourgeault, I.L., Atanackovic, J., LeBrun, J., Parpia, R., Rashid, A. and Winkup, J. (2010). *Immigrant Care Workers in Aging Societies: The Canadian Context and Experience*. Ottawa: Ontario Health Human Resource Research Network.

Brickner, R.K. and Straehle, C. (2010). The missing link: Gender, immigration policy and the live-in caregiver program in Canada. *Policy and Society*, 29, 309–320.

Buck, P.S. (1954). *My Several Worlds*. New York: Open Road.

Burrows, S. (2013). Precarious work, neo-liberalism and young people's experiences of employment in the Illawarra region. *Economic and Labour Relations Review*, 24(3), 380–396.

Calasanti, T. and King, N. (2015). Intersectionality and age. In J. Twigg and W. Martin (eds), *Routledge Handbook of Cultural Gerontology* (pp. 193–200). New York: Routledge.

Canadian Immigration News (2015, May). Philippines was top source country for new immigrants to Canada in 2014. *CIC News*. Retrieved from www.cicnews.com/2015/05/philippines-top-source-country-immigrants-canada-2014-055253.html.

Cangiano, A. (2014). Elder care and migrant labor in Europe: A demographic outlook. *Population and Development Review, 40*, 1131–1154.

CBC News (2010, April 26). Ontario won't regulate personal care workers. *CBC News*. Retrieved from www.cbc.ca/news/canada/toronto/ontario-won-t-regulate-personal-care-workers-1.907601.

Chatterjee, P. (2011). Progress patch, on health-worker crisis. *The Lancet, 377*, 456.

Creese, G. (2011). Government restructuring and settlement agencies in Vancouer: Bringing advocacy back. In C. Milligan and D. Conradson (eds), *Landscapes of Voluntarism: New Spaces of Health, Welfare and Governance*. Bristol: Policy Press.

Crenshaw, K. (1989). Demarginalizing the intersection of race and sex: A black feminist critique of antidiscrimination doctrine, feminist theory and antiracist politics. *University of Chicago Legal Forum, 140*, 139–167.

de Torres, S. (2002). *Understanding Persons of Phillippine Origin: A Primer for Rehabilitation Service Providers*. Phillippines: Center for International Rehabilitation Research Information and Exchange. Retrieved from http://cirrie.buffalo.edu/culture/monographs/philippines.php.

Dery, R. (2015, October 20). 10 changes coming to Canada's immigration system with a new government. *Canadim*. Retrieved from www.canadim.com/justin-trudeau-canadian-immigration.

Eckenwiler, L. (2014). Care worker migration, global health equity and ethical place-making. *Women's Studies International Forum, 47*, 213–222.

Faraday, F. (2014). Profiting from the precarious. Metcalf Foundation. Retrieved from http://metcalffoundation.com/wp-content/uploads/2014/04/Profiting-from-the-Precarious.pdf.

Federici, S. (2012). On elder care. *The Commoner, 15*, 235–261.

Few-Demo, A.L. (2014). Intersectionality as the "new" critical approach in feminist family studies: Evolving racial/ethnic feminisms and critical race theories. *Journal of Family Theory & Review, 6*, 169–183.

Fisher, T. (2006). Race, neoliberalism and "welfare reform" in Britain. *Social Justice, 33*(3), 54–65.

Freixas, A., Luque, B. and Reina, A. (2012). Critical feminist gerontology: In the back room of research. *Journal of Women & Aging, 24*, 44–58.

Ganti, T. (2014). Neoliberalism. *Annual Review of Anthropology, 43*, 89–104.

Gardiner Barber, P. and Bryan, C. (2012). Value plus plus: Housewifization and history in Philippine care migration. In P. Gardiner Barber and W. Lem (eds), *Migration in the 21st Century: Political Economy and Ethnography*. New York: Routledge.

Giles, W. and Arat-Koc, S. (1994). *Maid in the Market: Women's Paid Domestic Labour*. Halifax: Fernwood.

Government of Canada (2015). *I am a Live-in Caregiver: What Happens if I Lose my Job?* Ottawa: Citizen and Immigration Canada. Retrieved from www.cic.gc.ca/english/helpcentre/answer.asp?qnum=226&top=28.

Greenwood, R.M. (2008). Intersectional political consciousness: Appreciation for intragroup differences and solidarity in diverse groups. *Psychology of Women Quarterly, 32*, 36–47.

Guerrero, S.H. (2000). Gender and migration: Focus on Filipino women in international labor migration. *Review of Women's Studies, 10*(1–2), 275–298.

Gundzik, J.P. (2005, June 16). Blind debt in the Phillippines. *Asia Times*. Retrieved from www.atimes.com/atimes/Southeast_Asia/GF16Ae01.html.

Hennebry, J. and Preibisch, K. (2012). A model for managed migration? Re-examining best practices in Canada's seasonal agricultural worker program. *International Migration, 50*, 19–40.

Hoppania, H.-K. and Vaittinen, T. (2014). A household full of bodies: Neoliberalism, care and "the political." *Global Society, 29*(1), 70–88.

Joseph, G. (1996). Some implications of free trade on Canada's aging population. In G. Joseph (ed.), *Difficult Issues in Aging in Difficult Times*. Guelph: University of Guelph.

Joseph, G., Leach, B. and Turner, S. (2007). *Caring at a Distance: Working Women, Rural to Urban Migration and the Compassionate Care Challenge*. Ottawa: Status of Women Canada.

Kalleberg, A.L. (2013). Globalization and precarious work. *Contemporary Sociology: A Journal of Reviews, 42*(5), 700–706.

Keefe, J. (2011). *Supporting Caregivers and Caregiving in an Aging Canada*. Faces of Aging, Institute for Research on Public Policy (IRPP). Retrieved from www.rdc-cdr.ca/supporting-caregivers-and-caregiving-aging-canada.

Kelly, P., Park, S., de Leon, C. and Priest, J. (2011). *Profile of Live-in Caregiver Immigrants to Canada, 1993–2009*. Toronto Immigrant Employment Data Initiative (TIEDI). Toronto: York University.

Law Commission of Ontario (2010). *Vulnerable Workers and Precarious Work Consultation Paper*. Law Commission of Ontario. Retrieved from www.lco-cdo.org/vulnerable-workers-final-report.pdf.

Leach, B. (2013). Canada's migrants without history: Neoliberal immigration regimes and Trinidadian transnationalism. *International Migration, 51*(2), 32–45.

Lee, E. and Johnstone, M. (2013). Global inequities: A gender-based analysis of the Live-in Caregiver Program and the Kirogi Phenomenon in Canada. *Journal of Women and Social Work, 28*(4), 401–414.

Lero, D. and Joseph, G. (2007). *A Systematic Review of the Literature on Combining Work and Eldercare in Canada*. Guelph: University of Guelph.

Lister, R. (2007). Inclusive citizenship: Realizing the potential. *Citizenship Studies, 11*(1), 49–61.

Mahler, S.J., Chaudhuri, M. and Patil, V. (2015). Scaling intersectionality: Advancing feminist analysis of transnational families. *Sex Roles, 73*, 100–112.

Marchitelli, R. (2015, October 27). Parents of disabled woman say caregiver's lack of medical skills put daughter at risk. *Go Public*. Retrieved from www.cbc.ca/news/canada/parents-frustrated-caregiver-who-lied-gets-to-stay-1.3284362.

Migneault, J. (2015, November 27). 10 years of care puts family on verge of burnout. *Northern Life*. Sudbury, Canada. Retrieved from www.sudbury.com/local-news/10-years-of-care-puts-family-on-verge-of-burnout-259137.

Migrant Mothers Project (2015). *Policy Brief: Live in Caregiver Program*. Toronto, Faculty of Social Work, University of Toronto. Retrieved from www.migrantmothersproject.com/policy-briefs.

Ontario Human Rights Commission (2000). *Discrimination and Age: Human Rights Issues Facing Older Persons in Ontario*. Toronto: Ontario Human Rights Commission.

Piche, V., Pelleier, E. and Epale, D. (2006). *Identification of the Obstacles to the Ratification of the United Nations International Convention on the Protection of the Rights of all Migrant Workers and Members of their Families: The Canadian*

Case. United Nations Educational, Scientific and Cultural Organization. Retrieved from http://unesdoc.unesco.org/images/0014/001473/147310E.pdf.

Roberts, D.J. and Mahtani, M. (2010). Neoliberalizing race, racing neoliberalism: Placing "race" in neoliberal discourses. *Antipode*, 42(2), 248–257.

Roberts, S.E. (2014). *The Classifying Work of Immigrant Policies in Canada: A Critical Analysis of the Temporary Foreign Workers Program and Access to Settlement Services*. Master thesis. Toronto: University of Toronto.

Romanow, R.J. (2002). *Building on Values: The Future of Health Care in Canada— Final Report of the Commission on the Future of Health Care in Canada*. Ottawa: National Library of Canada.

Root, J., Gates-Gasse, E., Shields, J. and Bauder, H. (2014). *Discounting Immigrant Families: Neoliberalism and the Framing of Canadian Immigration Policy Change*. Toronto: Ryerson Centre for Immigration and Settlement.

Salami, B., Nelson, S., McGillis Hall, L., Muntaner, C. and Hawthorne, L. (2014). Workforce integration of Philippine-educated nurses who migrate to Canada through the live-in caregiver program. *Canadian Journal of Nursing Research*, 46(4), 65–82.

Salvador, R. (2015). *Migrant Workers and the Canadian Live-in Caregiver Program: The Impact on Multigenerational Family*. Master thesis. Kingston: Queens University.

Schwiter, K., Berndt, C. and Truong, J. (2015). Neoliberal austerity and the marketisation of elderly care. *Social & Cultural Geography*. Retrieved from www.tandfonline.com/doi/full/10.1080/14649365.2015.1059473.

Sher, J. (2015, July 15). Dr. Christopher Mackie slammed for pitting young vs. old. *London Free Press*. Retrieved from www.lfpress.com/2015/07/15/mackie-slammed-for-pitting-young-vs-old.

Standing, G. (2011). *The Precariat: The New Dangerous Class*. London: Bloomsbury Academic.

Tibe Bonifacio, G. and Angeles, V.S. (2010). Building communities through faith: Filipino Catholics in Philadelphia and Alberta. In G. Tibe Bonifacio and V. Angeles (eds), *Gender, Religion and Migration: Pathways of Integration*. Lanham, MD: Lexington Books.

Tungohan, E. (2015, November 23). Abuse and barriers increase under new caregiver program regulations. *Rabble.ca*. Retrieved from http://rabble.ca/news/2015/09/abuse-and-barriers-increase-under-new-caregiver-program-regulations.

Urbano, R. (2011). Global justice and the plight of Filipino domestic migrant workers. *Journal of Asian and African Studies*, 47(6), 605–619.

Valbuena, J. (2013). *Filipino Women Caring for your Health: But What do You Care?* Montreal: Montreal Serai. Retrieved from http://montrealserai.com/2013/06/23/filipino-women-caring-for-your-health-but-what-do-you-care.

Verbeeten, D., Astles, P. and Prada, G. (2015). *Understanding Health and Social Services for Seniors in Canada*. Ottawa: Conference Board of Canada.

9 Vision care services in long-term care facilities

Why are they overlooked?

Pamela Hawranik, Sandy Bell and Donnie McIntosh

Estimates of the prevalence of vision impairment vary depending on the definitions and the methodologies used, however statistics remain alarming. The Canadian National Institute for the Blind (CNIB) (2006) estimates that one in nine Canadians over 65 years develop irreversible vision loss and that this number increases to one in four adults over 80 years of age. Ninety-two percent of persons over 70 years of age wear glasses. An additional 18 percent also use a magnifying glass for reading or close work. Fourteen percent of individuals aged 70–74 years and 32 percent of those over 85 report difficulties seeing even with correctional devices (Tabloski, 2010). The CNIB (2006) predicts that these ratios will increase with the aging of the population.

Visual deficits accompany the aging process (Houde and Huff, 2003). Cataracts, macular degeneration, glaucoma, diabetic retinopathy and refractory issues, including presbyopia, comprise the most prevalent causes of vision deficits in seniors (Groessl et al., 2013; Stuen and Faye, 2003). These conditions, which are correctable and/or treatable, can have profound consequences for the independence of the older adult and can lead to falls, fractures, depression, social isolation, behavioral issues and can aggravate behaviors associated with cognitive impairment (Berger and Powell, 2008; LaGrow et al., 2006; Lin et al., 2013; Lopez et al., 2011; Rogers and Langa, 2010). In fact, older adults with vision loss enter nursing homes three years earlier than those with normal vision, have twice as many falls and are four times more likely to fracture a hip (Ham et al., 2007; National Coalition for Vision Health, 2011).

Older residents in nursing homes have a substantially higher prevalence of blindness and vision impairment than their community-dwelling counterparts. The Baltimore Nursing Home Survey (Tielsch et al., 2008) reported overall prevalence of blindness among people 80 years of age and older ranging from 2.4 to 3.7 times higher in the nursing home population than among those living in the community. However, the vision history of individuals who are admitted to long-term care is often not well-documented. Further, once admitted, a systematic or periodic vision examination does not necessarily occur unless a problem arises (Bell et al., 2006; Carcenac et al., 2009; Hawranik and Bell, 2007).

This chapter will highlight the state of vision care in long-term care facilities in Canada and internationally. The implementation and evaluation of a vision care program in a personal care home will be described with a discussion of the barriers and facilitators to improving vision care for older adults in these facilities. Long-term care facilities will be a term used generally to describe institutions that provide 24-hour activity of daily living and nursing care to adults 65 years and older. In some jurisdictions, these facilities are called "nursing homes" or "personal care homes."

The state of vision care in long-term care facilities

A high prevalence of visual problems exist in older adults who reside in institutions. The majority of the vision impairment observed in long-term care facilities stems from treatable visual problems, such as refractive errors and cataracts (Carcenac et al., 2009; Wang et al., 2000). The Baltimore Eye survey (Rahmani et al., 1996) and the Blue Mountains Study (Wang et al., 2000) reported consistent findings that cataracts were the predominant cause of the high prevalence of visual impairment in people 75 years and older.

Poor vision is related to impaired balance and increased risk for falling (Black and Wood, 2005; Cox et al., 2005a). A small number of studies have identified a relationship between vision loss and an increased risk of hip fractures (Chew et al., 2010; Ivers et al., 2003; Public Health Agency of Canada, 2005). Some of this research has suggested that simple refractory alterations and cataract surgery can impact positively on falls and fractures in people over 65 years of age (Harwood et al., 2005). Schwartz et al. (2005) found that cataract surgery significantly improved postural stability, leading to a reduced risk of falling in a sample of older adults.

Vision has a major impact on the individual's dependency level with serious and costly consequences if undetected and untreated. Intuitively, it is accepted that vision can affect one's independence, mobility and behaviors, and, when combined with other chronic illnesses, can have an even more serious effect on that individual's dependency level. And yet, there appears to be minimal attention paid to the vision sensory function by staff, the older adults themselves and family members.

Few studies have evaluated in a systematic fashion the state of vision care services in long-term care facilities. Kergoat et al. (2014) distributed a questionnaire to long-term care facilities in Quebec to evaluate the perceived needs and availability of eye care services. The questionnaire was completed by a member of staff identified by the facility as the person most suitable to answer the questions. There were 196 facilities out of 428 facilities that responded. Seventy percent of the facilities indicated that the majority of their residents wore glasses and 45 percent reported that a substantial portion of their residents received treatment for their eyes. An interesting finding was that upon admission, 84 percent of the facilities indicated they ask questions about the individual's oculovisual health, but did not offer any formal screening. A "good" proportion (a term used in Kergoat et al., 2014) of the respondents reported that there were no barriers to eye care services in their institution. However, from the survey results, limited services were offered and limited numbers of residents did obtain eye care services. The respondents reported that for those who had barriers to vision care, lack of ability to cooperate for an eye exam and lack of professionals to offer the services were most frequently cited. The results of Kergoat and colleagues' study reflected similar results found in two province-wide surveys conducted by Hawranik and Bell (2014a, 2014b).

The Manitoba survey (Hawranik and Bell, 2014b) of 84 rural facilities outside of Winnipeg revealed findings similar to the Quebec study (Kergoat et al., 2014) . In the Manitoba survey, six out of the 56 facilities that responded indicated they had a policy/procedure for vision care services. However, the policies they identified were listed as "cleaning of glasses," "making sure the resident was wearing their glasses" and "labelling of glasses." When asked why they did not have a policy, the most frequent reasons reported were "has not been discussed" and "no staff or resources available to implement a policy." No facility conducted vision screening. A combination of the resident, family and nurse were the most frequently mentioned as the individuals responsible for determining whether a resident needed to obtain vision testing and follow-up. The staff did identify barriers to seeking vision care services, with the most frequently mentioned as limited mobility of the resident, transportation difficulties, no services nearby and vision testing and treatment being unnecessary. Certainly the transportation and lack of available services would be relevant since the facilities were located in rural communities.

A similar survey in the province of Alberta was conducted (Hawranik and Bell, 2014a) to identify the nature of vision care services provided in long-term care facilities throughout the province. Out of 261 eligible facilities, 79 completed the survey. Thirty-five of the facilities included vision questions in their falls risk assessment tool. More than half of the facilities (55 percent) indicated they did not have a nursing procedure/policy/best practice guideline for the care of vision aides, with only 11 percent indicating they did. Only 21 percent had a policy/procedure/practice guideline on vision care services. Three of the facilities had an eye care specialist provide services on-site. Similar to the Manitoba study, the most frequently identified reasons for not having a vision care policy/procedure/practice guideline were "no staff or resources to implement this" and "has not been discussed." As in the Manitoba study (Hawranik and Bell, 2014b), 27 (34 percent) of the facilities indicated that the primary responsibility for obtaining vision care services is a combination of the nurse, resident and family. The most frequent barriers to obtaining vision care services were limited mobility, arranging transportation and the resident or family not considering vision testing and intervention important.

The three surveys illustrate that basic prevention and treatment of vision problems occur to a very limited extent in long-term care facilities. The results from these three Canadian provinces are not unique to Canada. A study in the Netherlands found that upon reviewing the medical records of nursing home residents, "there was no special attention being paid to vision problems in the nursing homes" (Sinoo et al., 2012, p. 1917). Minimal recording of visual problems was seen in the medical records. No significant difference was found in whether information was recorded when residents had normal vision as compared to residents with low vision or blindness. Professional visits by eye care providers to the nursing homes tended not to occur.

A survey of vision care services in 45 participating long-term care homes in Aberdeen, Scotland, revealed a similar lack of understanding and application of quality practice in the area of vision care services (Bell et al., 2011). Only one of the 45 homes in the sample had a documented policy for vision care services. While vision care services are made available by a private service provider, it remains the responsibility of the resident to articulate visual problems or, alternatively, it is left to staff to note changes in behavior and make the necessary referral. Further, little attention was paid to the causes of falls or any relationship between vision impairment and falling.

Residents in long-term care settings are dependent upon their caregivers for their care. They may not be aware of their deteriorating vision and may not have the cognitive and functional ability to determine whether they need a vision assessment, how to make necessary appointments, arrange for the transportation, attend the appointment, agree to recommended intervention and then comply with the recommended treatment. Further, the reasons indicated in the three Canadian surveys for a lack of vision care policy or procedures were lack of resources to conduct screening or provide any assistance with referral and follow-up.

The authors of this chapter decided to challenge the previous research and introduce an intervention program that provided vision care services to a long-term care facility. An evaluation of that program was also conducted. This next section will briefly describe the program and the evaluation that took place to examine the validity of a vision screening tool and the feasibility of a vision care program.

The vision care intervention program

The program was called the Focus on Falls Prevention Project and is described in detail in a previously published paper (Bell et al., 2011). The project occurred over a one-year period and was funded by Manitoba Health and Misericordia Health Centre. The project took place on a 100-bed personal care home in Misericordia Health Centre. The facility was located in a major urban centre and housed the Eye Care Centre of Excellence, the largest comprehensive surgical and treatment eye care centre in Western

Canada. Despite the location of the personal care home in this centre, the residents did not have access to the vision care services provided by the Centre of Excellence.

In order to participate in the program, the participants had to be residents of the personal care home and 65 years or older. The project involved the use of the Vision Screening Kit by a registered nurse, referral to the appropriate healthcare or vision care provider, arrangements for the transportation to the appropriate eye care provider and scheduled recommended interventions with appropriate follow-up. Interventions included cataract surgery, new eyeglass prescription, eye drop prescription, glaucoma treatment or referral to agencies such as the CNIB. Costs related to the treatments were covered by the project, relieving the individual resident of expenses for the needed interventions. Special medical records were created for the nurse to record the information from the screening, the recommendations and the effects of the intervention.

The Vision Screening Kit

The Vision Screening Kit was used for the screening in the Focus on Falls Prevention Project with its validity being tested in the evaluation study. The kit was based on the World Health Organization Low Vision Kit (Carnicelli, 2001; Keeffe et al., 1996; Nottle et al., 2000). The kit was used in a joint initiative between the Royal Victorian Eye and Ear Hospital and the Centre for Eye Research Australia to facilitate access to regular vision screening for people 65 years and older. The kit has been used on seniors who reside in aged care facilities and in the community. It has also been successful in detecting vision loss in individuals with cognitive impairment. The tool was adapted to meet North American vision assessment conversions.

The kit consists of letter "E" vision cards for testing distance vision and near vision, a pinhole mask and an instruction booklet with vision testing forms. The purpose of the kit is to detect the presence of vision loss that may affect the person's day-to-day activities (Carnicelli, 2001). Specific visual disorders cannot be identified. The kit also contains an algorithm that directs the tester, depending upon the results, to the most appropriate eye care provider—an optician, optometrist or ophthalmologist. The screening using the tool takes approximately ten minutes by a trained individual. No reliability or validity data was available on the kit at the time of the intervention program.

The evaluation of the vision care intervention program

The purpose of the evaluation was to identify the prevalence of vision disorders from the medical records and the screening, test the validity of the vision screening kit and determine whether the Focus on Falls Prevention program did affect falls and fractures.

For the purposes of the study, vision care services were defined as vision screening, vision assessment, referral, intervention and follow-up to the intervention. It was a retrospective pre- and post-measurement study. A pre-test or baseline measurement of the participants' characteristics was obtained, including such information as demographic characteristics, date of last eye examination and use of prescription lens. Additional information from the medical records was collected by the nurse on certain indicators three months before and three months after the intervention, such as Minimum Data Set (MDS) data on medications, diagnoses and number of falls and fractures.

Purposive sampling of older adults who had agreed to participate in the Focus on Falls Prevention program were approached for the study. Exclusion criteria were those residents whose dependency level was so high that they were unable to be transported for screening and intervention; had advanced dementia; or were experiencing an acute illness at the time scheduled for the screening.

A registered nurse conducted the screening on the participants using the vision screening kit. The participants were then referred to the optometrist for assessment. The optometrist, who had agreed to participate in the study, did not know the screening results from the nurse (the results of vision loss testing and the algorithm outcome). The individual received the necessary referral recommended by the optometrist.

The sample consisted of 92 residents. Inconsistent and incomplete information was discovered in the medical records. Only 18 (19 percent) of the records indicated the resident had a vision diagnosis at the time of their admission to the facility. However, 69 (75 percent) of the charts had an entry that the resident wore glasses. In 72 (78 percent) of the charts, there was no recorded data of the last eye examination. Only 19 (20 percent) of the records indicated that the resident had fallen in the past three months.

As mentioned earlier, the screening tool identifies whether there is vision loss and to whom a referral should be made. Vision loss was identified in 77 of the 92 residents by the nurse. The optometrist, who was not made aware of the results from the screening, found 79 of the residents had vision loss. The strength of agreement between the nurse's identification of vision loss and the optometrist's was 97.5 percent. The algorithm in the vision kit enabled the nurse to determine to whom to refer the resident. The nurse determined that 52 of the residents should be referred for ophthalmology and 25 for optometry, while the optometrist identified 49 residents for ophthalmology and 28 for optometry. Using Kappa, the strength of agreement between the nurse's referral algorithm and the optometrist's determination was .799 (p < .000), an excellent strength of association.

Although 92 residents agreed to be screened, not all received the recommended treatment(s). It was determined by the optometrist that 55 out of the 92 participants required and would benefit from some form of intervention and were subsequently referred to an ophthalmologist, physician, optician or the CNIB. However, only 17 agreed to accept the intervention.

The type of care they received included new lens prescription; cataract surgery; vitamin prescription; application of hot compresses; and referral to the CNIB for visual aids.

There were a number of reasons for the individuals not accepting the referral or obtaining the recommended treatment (n=38 out of the 55 who were referred)—one individual passed away during the study period before they obtained the treatment; eight did not attend for a number of reasons, including being unable to obtain the necessary treatment due to mobility and transfer difficulties; and 29 refused to receive any treatment.

Reasons for refusal of the referral and treatment were provided by a number of the residents and family members. The most common reasons given included: "don't use vision much in a nursing home so I don't need the treatment" and "it won't make any difference." In another case, the family and resident stated "she is too old." In another situation, the family indicated they felt the resident could read well enough and did not need new glasses.

Additional statistical analysis was conducted to detect differences between those residents who received the intervention (n=17) and those who either refused or did not receive the treatment (n=38). No statistically significant differences were found between these two groups before they received the intervention, in terms of age, gender, diagnoses, cognitive status, depression, balance or length of time in the facility. However, interesting data emerged on the differences in falls and fractures between those who received intervention compared to those who did not receive the intervention due to either refusal or inability to obtain the intervention.

No falls or fractures occurred in the group that received intervention for the subsequent three-month period. In the group that did not receive the intervention (n=38), falls occurred in 18 of the residents. Out of the 18 residents, eight residents experienced a fracture from a fall. Three deaths occurred from resultant hip fractures.

The findings of the study do reflect the past and current research and documentation on the lack of attention to vision care in long-term care facilities. However, the evaluation results do hold potential for feasible and relevant practice and policy changes.

Discussion

The lack of policy on vision care in long-term care facilities illustrates the low priority that is placed on vision and its importance to many dimensions of an individual's quality of life and independence.

In the evaluation study, there was a substantial number of residents who did not accept a referral or who followed through with the referral but refused the recommended treatment. This was surprising to the researchers. Perhaps the residents' perceptions reflected those of the general population in that they did not see a need for an eye examination. A recent survey by the

Canadian Association of Optometrists found that 57 percent of Canadians believe eye examinations are only necessary for people who are experiencing eye problems (CNIB, 2015). Only 69 percent of Canadians actually do get their eyes checked every two years by an optometrist. Reasons cited for not visiting an optometrist in the survey included: don't have any eye problems; no insurance coverage; and lack of time (Canadian Association of Optometrists, 2007). And, yet, disorders such as cataracts and glaucoma occur insidiously and gradually.

Some of the statements by the older adults and their families reflected the belief that they are able to read and therefore do not need new lenses. As seen in the evaluation study, one of the reasons for not accepting the recommended intervention was that decreased sight was considered a natural part of aging. This lack of awareness and understanding of vision loss was mentioned by the residents and family members. In one case, an ophthalmologist refused to provide the intervention stating "the resident is in a nursing home and does not use his eyes much." In another Canadian study (Gold et al., 2006), the older adult participants reported that eye care professionals, mainly ophthalmologists, commonly told them that "nothing more can be done" once it was determined that their vision loss could not be reversed by medication or surgery. This same attitude was also reported in an Australian study (Pollard et al., 2003) and a Quebec study (Gresset et al., 2005).

A remarkable and yet consistent finding was the inadequate recording in the medical records of the individual's vision history. An American study (Owsley et al., 2007) found that 66 percent of resident records had no information about an eye examination. In a study conducted in the Netherlands (Sinoo et al., 2012), 46 percent of the participating residents were referred to an ophthalmologist or to a rehabilitation centre. In a significant number of cases, no information on visual problems was reported in the resident's medical records. Unfortunately, this was the case in the evaluation study. It was reported that some vision questions were asked at the time of admission and yet this information was not recorded.

The responsibility of vision care and obtaining the necessary vision care services tends to be left to the older adult or their family/friend to identify that a problem exists and conduct the subsequent appointments and activities that may be needed. It is well-documented in long-term care facilities there is a high prevalence of visual problems and neurodegenerative diseases that can affect cognition and communication, making it difficult for the residents to express or recognize their visual problems (Kergoat et al., 2014). Lack of transportation and companion availability to accompany the nursing home resident to the appointments may be influential factors in the resident not receiving screening and intervention (Cox et al., 2005b; Friedman et al., 2005).

The reasons cited for not having a policy or not implementing any meaningful assessment or follow-up reflect not only a lack of knowledge but ageist beliefs of staff and decision makers. There may be an assumption that the effort to screen or arrange for vision appointments is not worthwhile given the need to coordinate and facilitate vision care. Cognitive impairment also seemed to become a reason for not screening for vision impairment, and that the older adult would not cooperate or would not benefit from vision care (Kergoat et al., 2014).

The lack of policies and procedures related to vision care in long-term care facilities was prevalent. Similar reasons for the lack of policy were reported in all three Canadian surveys, namely a lack of resources. Without direction from administrators and researchers, vision problems in older adults in long-term care facilities will continue to go undetected, leading to increasing dependency needs when decline could be delayed or, in some cases, preventing certain conditions as a result of vision loss.

At the macro level, there are no guidelines or standards that provide direction to staff to include vision as a risk factor for falls. Both the Canadian Ophthalmological Society and the Canadian Association of Optometrists have developed clinical practice guidelines and professional standards for competency. However, Canada has not yet developed a national plan or policy standards to govern vision care, except for cataract surgery wait times (Muzychka, 2009), despite the fact that it was instrumental in the passage of the Global Initiative for the Elimination of Avoidable Blindness (Resolution 56.26) at the World Health Assembly in 2003 (World Health Organization, 2006). This resolution called on member states to develop a national plan for blindness prevention by 2005.

Implications/recommendations for policy

Recommendations for changes to attitudes, knowledge, behavior and policy and practice are easily identified. Many facilities are now developing "moving in agreements" which review policies and expectations of the facility and the resident/family caregivers. These require specified assessments using validated tools such as falls risk and physical assessment. Vision assessment can be included in the agreement.

The screening tool took approximately ten minutes for the registered nurse to administer. The tool was found to be highly valid. Vision screening could be done by the nurse at the time of admission to the facility and then every other year.

Many older adults are concerned about the costs of vision care. Most provincial health plans will cover expenses related to an optometrist visit and eyeglasses prescription bi-annually. Discussion with the older adult on the health plan in their jurisdiction may facilitate their decision to obtain screening and treatment as needed.

One of the frequently mentioned reasons for staff not implementing a vision policy or conducting screening was inadequate resources. If the facility is unwilling to facilitate testing by nurses, perhaps volunteers could be trained in using this vision screening kit.

Vision is taken for granted and the gradual and insidious deterioration that can occur goes unnoticed. Greater public health promotion of aging changes and vision disorders is needed.

Education campaigns about vision health must include all Canadians, not only seniors. Health curricula for healthcare providers may be one method of increasing the awareness and knowledge of these professionals. Content to address ageism is important to include. Linkages between vision and the consequences of untreated vision disorders must be explicitly incorporated in the curriculum.

There is no national strategy on vision health. National standards on vision health with collaborative planning at the provincial and national levels may help to educate the public and provide greater direction on creating policy for all age groups in the area of prevention and treatment of vision disorders.

Rural areas of Canada continue to experience shortages of eye care specialists and accessibility to such resources. Strategies and policy to support vision screening in long-term facilities, by the use of the vision screening kit, could help in delaying and treating vision disorders and leading to direct referrals to the most appropriate eye care specialist.

Residents in the long-term care setting are dependent upon their caregivers for their care. Assessing the visual needs and supporting older adults and their families as they seek appropriate vision care is important. It is the right of the older person in the long-term care setting to receive high-quality care, a sense of security and belonging and a sense of feeling valued.

Conclusion

The research on vision care of older adults is consistent in its findings on the lack of attention in detecting and treating visual impairment. The high costs of vision loss and falls and fractures in the elderly is well-documented in a number of major reports, and yet across Canada and other parts of the world, minimal attention is given to establishing standards and practice guidelines for services. The growing aging population will only escalate healthcare costs and lead to greater dependency in older adults if policies and practices are not put into place. Previous studies have not only reported on the lack of attention from the formal system to deal with vision, aging and falls, but also the need for education of all parties not to automatically accept limitations in elderly individuals as normal aging changes, and to enhance the quality of life of seniors by offering interventions in areas that will readily improve their health.

References

Bell, S., Briggs. S., Grant, I. and Hawranik, P. (2006). *Eyes on the Elderly: A Study of Vision Care Services in Long-Term Care Homes in Canada and Scotland.* Unpublished report.

Bell, S., Hawranik, P. and McCormac, K. (2011). Focus on falls prevention: A quality improvement initiative. *Insight: Research and Practice in Visual Impairment and Blindness*, 4(3), 133–138.

Berger, S. and Powell, F. (2008). The association between low vision and function. *Journal of Aging and Health*, 20, 504–525.

Black, A. and Wood, J. (2005). Vision and falls. *Clinical Exp Optometry*, 88, 212–222.

Canadian Association of Optometrists (2007). Eye health awareness: Eye-opening stats about seniors. *Canadian Healthcare Manager*, 14(5), 26.

Canadian National Institute for the Blind (CNIB). (2006). Vision loss "major health concern" for Albertans: Poll. Retrieved from www.cnib.ca/en/about/Publications/newsletters/Insight/122006/pages/research.aspx.

Canadian National Institute for the Blind (CNIB). (2015). *Canadians Leave Themselves at Risk for Detectable Eye Disease: Cao Survey*. Retrieved from www.cnib.ca/en/research/news/CAO-survey-0208/Pages/default.aspx.

Carcenac, G., Herard, M.-E., Kergoat, M., Lajeunesse, Y., Champoux, N., Barauskas, A. and Kergoat, H. (2009). Assessment of visual function in institutionalized elderly patients. *Journal of the American Medical Directors Association*, 10(1), 45–49.

Carnicelli, A. (2001). *Vision Screening for Older People: A Joint Initiative Between the Royal Victoria Eye and Ear Hospital and the Centre for Eye Research Australia*. Australia: Royal Victoria Eye and Ear Hospital and the Centre for Eye Research Australia.

Chew, F., Yong, C., Mas, A. and Tajunisah, I. (2010). The association between various visual function tests and low fragility hip fractures among the elderly: A Malaysian experience. *Age & Ageing*, 39(2), 239–245.

Cox, A., Blaikie, A., MacEwen, C., Jones, D., Thompson, K., Holding, D., Sharma, T., Miller, S., Dobson, S. and Sanders, R. (2005a). Optometric and ophthalmic contact in elderly hip fracture patients with visual impairment. *Ophthalmology Physiology Optometry*, 25, 357–362.

Cox, A., Blaikie, A., MacEwen, C., Jones, D., Thompson, K., Holding, D., Sharma, T., Miller, S., Dobson, S. and Sanders, R. (2005b). Visual impairment in elder patients with hip fracture: Causes and associations. *Eye*, 19, 652–656.

Friedman, D., Munoz, B., Roche, K., Massof, R., Broman, A. and West, S. (2005). Poor uptake of cataract surgery in nursing home residents: The Salisbury eye evaluation in nursing home groups study. *Archives of Ophthalmology*, 123(11), 1581–1587.

Gold, D., Zuvela, B. and Hodge, W. (2006). Perspectives on low vision service in Canada: A pilot study. *Canadian Journal of Ophthalmology*, 41(3), 348–354.

Gresset, J., Jalbert, Y. and Gauthier, M. (2005). Elderly persons confronted with visual loss and long waiting lists: How do they react? *International Congress Series*, 1282, 143–146.

Groessl, E., Liu, M., Sklar, S., Tally, R., Kaplan, R. and Ganiats, T. (2013). Measuring the impact of cataract surgery on generic and vision-specific quality of life. *Quality of Life Research*, 22(6), 1405–1414.

Ham, R., Sloane, P., Warshaw, G., Bernard, M. and Flaherty, E. (2007). *Primary Care Geriatrics: A Case-based Approach* (5th edn). Philadelphia, PN: Mosby Elsevier.

Harwood, R., Foos, A., Osborn, F., Gregson, R., Zaman, A. and Masud, T. (2005). Falls and health status in elderly women following eye cataract surgery: A randomized controlled trial. *British Journal of Ophthalmology*, 89, 53–59.

Hawranik, P. and Bell, S. (2007). Vision care in long-term care facilities: An overlooked need. *Canadian Journal of Geriatrics*, 10(3), supplement, 15–18.

Hawranik, P. and Bell, S. (2014a). *A Survey of Vision Care Services Provided in Long-term Care Facilities in Alberta. Final Report.* Unpublished.

Hawranik, P. and Bell, S. (2014b). *A Survey of Vision Care Services Provided in Personal care Homes in Rural Manitoba. Final Report.* Unpublished.

Houde, S. and Huff, M. (2003). Age-related vision loss in older adults. *Journal of Gerontological Nursing*, 4, 25–32.

Ivers, R., Optom, B., Cumming, R., Mitchell, P., Simpson, J. and Peduto, A. (2003). Visual risk factors for hip fractures in older people. *Journal of American Geriatrics Society*, 51, 356–363.

Keeffe, J., Lovie-Kitchin, J., MacLean, H. and Taylor, H. (1996). A simplified screening test for identifying people with low vision in developing countries. *Bulletin of the World Health Organization*, 74(5), 525–532.

Kergoat, H., Boisjoly, H., Freeman, E., Monette, J., Roy, S. and Kergoat, M. (2014). The perceived needs and availability of eye care services for older adults in long-term care facilities. *Canadian Geriatrics Journal*, 17(3), 108–113.

LaGrow, S., Robertson, M., Campbell, A., Clarke, G. and Kerse, N. (2006). Reducing hazard related falls in people 75 years and older with significant visual impairment: How did a successful program work? *Injury Prevention*, 12(5): 296–301.

Lin, E., Yaffe, K., Xia, J., Xuc, Q., Harris, T., Purchase-Helzner, E. and Simonsick, E. (2013). Hearing loss and cognitive decline in older adults. *Journal of the American Medical Association*, 173, 293–299.

Lopez, D., McCaul, K. Hankey, G., Norman, P., Almeida, O., Dobson, A. and Flicker, L. (2011). Falls, injuries from falls, health related quality of life and morality in older adults with vision and hearing impairment: Is there a gender difference? *Maturitas*, 69, 359–364.

Muzychka, M. (2009). *Environmental Scan of Vision Health and Vision Loss in the Provinces and Territories of Canada.* National Coalition for Vision Health. Ottawa, Ontario.

National Coalition for Vision Health (2011). *Vision Loss in Canada 2011.* Retrieved from www.cos-sco.ca/wp-content/uploads/2012/09/VisionLossinCanada_e.pdf.

Nottle, H., McCarty, C., Hassell, J. and Keeffe, J. (2000). Detection of vision impairment in people admitted to aged care assessment centres. *Clinical and Experimental Ophthalmology*, 28, 162–164.

Owsley, C., McGwin, G., Scilley, K., Meek, G., Dyer, A. and Seker, D. (2007). The visual status of older persons residing in nursing homes. *Archives of Ophthalmology*, 125(7), 925–930.

Pollard, T., Simpson, J., Lamoureux, E. and Keeffe, J. (2003). Barriers to accessing low vision services. *Ophthalmic and Physiological Optics*, 23, 321–327.

Public Health Agency of Canada (2005). *Inventory of Fall Prevention Initiatives in Canada—2005.* Ottawa, ON: Division of Aging and Seniors, Public Health Agency of Canada.

Rahmani, B., Tielsch, J., Katz, J., Gottsch, J., Quigley, H., Javitt, J. and Sommer, A. (1996). The cause-specific prevalence of visual impairment in an urban population: The Baltimore eye survey. *Ophthalmology*, 103(11), 1721–1726.

Rogers, M. and Langa, K. (2010). Untreated poor vision: A contributing factor to late-life dementia. *American Journal of Epidemiology, 171*, 728–735.

Schwartz, S., Segal, O., Barkana, Y., Schwesig, R., Avni, I. and Morad, Y. (2005). The effect of cataract surgery on postural control. *Investigative Ophthalmology & Visual Science, 46*(5), 920–924.

Sinoo, M., Kort, H. and Duijnstee, M. (2012). Visual functioning in nursing home residents: Information in client records. *Journal of Clinical Nursing, 21*, 1913–1921.

Stuen, C. and Faye, E. (2003). Vision loss: Normal and not normal changes among older adults. *Generations, 27*, 8–14.

Tabloski, P. (2010). *Gerontological Nursing* (2nd edn). Upper Saddle River, NJ: Pearson Education.

Tielsch, J., Javitt, J., Coleman, A., Katz, J. and Sommer, A. (2008). The prevalence of blindness and visual impairment among nursing home residents in Baltimore. *New England Journal of Medicine, 332*(18), 1205–1209.

Wang, J., Foran, S. and Mitchell, P. (2000). Age-specific prevalence and causes of bilateral and unilateral visual impairment in older Australians: The Blue Mountains Eye Study. Clinical & *Experimental Ophthalmology, 28*, 268–273.

World Health Organization (2006). *WHO Monitoring Committee for the Elimination of Avoidable Blindness. Report of the First Meeting.* Geneva: World Health Organization.

Section 3

Aging and economics

10 When healthcare is delivered in your home, will you need to make economic trade-offs?

Lee Anne Davies, John P. Hirdes and Roger Mannell

Poverty means that an individual's legitimate needs cannot be met (Williamson, 2000). An increasing number of people in Canada experiencing health issues are facing a loss of economic security, left each day to decide between necessities such as heat or groceries (Raphael, 2002). For some, the situation becomes extreme, resulting in loss of key financial assets, income sources and even impending personal bankruptcy (Sharratt, 2015). Yet, Canada is a country with a national social safety net and universal healthcare programs that are intended to meet the needs of its residents, regardless of ability to pay. This gap between assumed availability of services and actual experience indicates that existing programs do not keep all residents immune from poverty.

Poverty can be hidden and may not be self-identified. Social inequalities such as the wide range of life expectancies between the least and the most materially deprived areas in Canada provide some insight into factors associated with poverty (Auger et al., 2010). As recent as the 1960s, Canada introduced policy that resulted in a decline in poverty levels and an improvement in health outcomes for those in lower income brackets (MacDonald et al., 2011). Universal healthcare and social infrastructures resulted, citizens benefited and Canadians were proud of the equality of access and treatment. However, very little improvement in poverty levels has been achieved since the mid-1990s (Bryant et al., 2011; Raphael, 2007). At the same time, the Canadian population is undergoing dramatic change due to rapid aging. In order to further reduce poverty levels, a readjustment of policy, program delivery and their supporting infrastructures is needed. This can be done most effectively through a better understanding of the characteristics of those most at risk of poverty in the aging Canadian population. Using rigorous scientific approaches, those most at risk of making economic trade-offs and associated factors can be best understood by examining their health outcomes and quality of life.

Many studies have examined seniors' poverty. Mainly for policy purposes, monetary measures, typically income, are often used to assess seniors' poverty, but these measures have a number of important limitations (Nolan and Whelan, 2010; Szanton et al., 2010). Financial information is both difficult to obtain because of its personal nature (Esser and Palme, 2010; Lawton et al., 1999; Lindeboom et al., 2002) and often inaccurate due to the low levels of financial literacy in the general population (Lusardi and Mitchell, 2009). Those attempting to improve the accuracy of financial reporting have avoided financial calculations and instead measured relative poverty or affluence based on people's perceptions. However, this approach is also unsatisfactory because it is confounded by people having different reference groups and unique life course experiences (Butterworth et al., 2009; Richmond and Ross, 2008; Sachs-Erricsson et al., 2009; Szanton et al., 2008; Whelan et al., 2001). In other words, individuals may not self-identify as living in poverty because their family and peer group share a similar lifestyle and everyone "manages."

Older persons present a greater challenge in measuring poverty due to their willingness to use their wealth (even the ownership of modest assets such as inexpensive jewellery are considered wealth) to supplement their income shortfalls. Consequently, it is more difficult to measure poverty when there is no paid workforce income in a cohort with an age range beginning at 55 and extending beyond 100 and is primarily retired. Those living on a fixed income in retirement try to avoid poverty by pawning valuables, thereby diminishing personal wealth in order to increase available cash (Brown, 1991; Haveman et al., 2006; Hyde et al., 2004). For most, this is a short-term option, limited by the availability of assets to pawn, market interest in their assets and functional ability to complete a pawning transaction. Unfortunately, this approach may delay identification of income inadequacies until a personal crisis is disclosed.

Deprivation measures offer suitable alternatives to income and other monetary indicators (Butterworth et al., 2009; Sachs-Erricsson et al., 2009; Szanton et al., 2008; Whelan et al., 2001). These types of non-monetary measures improve the understanding of cash flow realities faced by individuals, regardless of their household wealth levels. This approach is especially useful in comparing across jurisdictions, locally, nationally and internationally, because income and wealth information is location-sensitive, as are appreciation and depreciation rates of many assets (Chiriboga et al., 2002; Rappaport and Siegel, 2009). Deprivation measures can include risks such as a failure to participate in supportive areas of life or of material deprivation (Goodridge et al., 2011; Nolan and Whelan, 2010). The well-being of "deprived" populations is often jeopardized (Jariah et al., 2006; Ross et al., 2000) by poor nutrition, diminished physical and mental health, inadequate shelter and social isolation. These populations experience higher rates of mortality (Hirdes and Forbes, 1989; Saunders and Adelman, 2006).

Canada's home care programs offer a unique opportunity to examine poverty risks in an older population. Individuals who are experiencing health issues and receiving healthcare services while continuing to live in their private homes are required to continue managing their day-to-day living environment. Daily activities such as buying groceries, making meals, paying bills and other duties in addition to caring for the person who is ill must continue. Risks of additional expenses and lost income are heightened. Although healthcare is universal in Canada, there are jurisdictional differences for reasons such as local policy, administration or population differences.

The authority for home care services lies with each of Canada's 13 provinces and territories (Health Canada, 2011). This results in wide variations of available services by province or territory. Although all will provide some level of nursing services, the number of hours of support and type of services offered will vary widely. Coverage for many other services such as homemaking, personal care and oxygen may range from unfunded through to fully funded based on assessed level of need. However, the assessed level eligible for public funding may still be insufficient to meet the care needs of the individual. Consequently, the purchasing of private services or an increased reliance on informal supports is required. Canada's system of health and social program may not meet the needs of this aging population, placing them increasingly at risk of poverty.

The development of a profile of those who are making economic trade-offs, and consequently are "deprived" to some extent, using non-monetary indicators may provide clearer insight into who is at risk. Information about the health status, social networks and demographics of older adults in home care will help determine where policy and program gaps exist. The current analysis is based on a unique database resulting from the administration of the interRAI Resident Assessment Instrument for Home Care (RAI-HC) (Carpenter and Hirdes, 2013; Gray et al., 2009; Hirdes, 2006; Morris et al., 1997). No published research, to the best of our knowledge, has utilized such a robust and multi-disciplinary database in order to better understand the characteristics of the aging poor. The current study provides the opportunity to identify risk factors for poverty, even for those people whose income is above standard cut-off points.

Approach

Data source

Data for this study came from home care assessment results using the 2002 Canadian version of the RAI-HC. A secondary analysis using data from the RAI-HC was completed for the Winnipeg Regional Health Authority (WRHA) and the provinces of Nova Scotia (NS) and Ontario (ON). These bi-annual assessments collect multi-dimensional data, including personal demographics, referral and discharge information, behavior patterns, informal support services, disease diagnosis, health conditions and environmental characteristics (Soldato et al., 2008). Observations and information are entered into the assessment considering the person's status over a three-day period with some exceptions, such as treatments that are measured over a seven-day period (Armstrong et al., 2010). Trained assessors (usually nurses or social workers) complete these assessments using clinical judgment to consider all sources of information available. Studies have demonstrated the strong inter-rater reliability and validity of the RAI-HC assessment protocol (Hawes et al., 2007; Hirdes et al., 2008).

The study population

Adult residents of Canada who have received publicly funded, long-stay home care services in the province of Nova Scotia, Ontario and from the WRHA are examined. There are slight differences in the services available in each provincial jurisdiction. Additional services can be purchased privately, but these are not tracked on the RAI-HC assessment.

A total of 935,053 assessments were available from the secured RAI-HC database at the University of Waterloo. Data are provided through agreements with the Canadian Institute for Health Information (CIHI) and the WRHA. The assessment data were collected from 2001 through to 2010, but not all regions provided data for every year. Since multiple records may exist for specific individuals who are reassessed over time, this study used only the first assessment record for those clients age 55 and over.

Missing data are a common problem in public health studies (Raghunathan, 2004) and in administrative databases (Nathan and Pawlik, 2007). In the database used for this study, data were missing for 9.1 percent (n=34,444) of the sample assessment records for the dependent variable. All but one client with missing data were from Ontario because the data warehouse did not have the automated routines to exclude observations with missing data during the initial years of implementation.

Measures

Description of the dependent variable

The assessor responds to a single trade-off question with a yes or no: "Because of limited funds, during the last month, client made trade-offs among purchasing any of the following: prescribed medications, sufficient home heat, necessary physician care, adequate food, home care." The assessor is directed to respond with a "yes" if trade-offs for the necessities specified are being made, regardless of how money is being used by the household. This approach is consistent with other studies probing material hardships or trade-offs (Butterworth et al., 2009; Sachs-Erricsson et al., 2009; Szanton et al., 2008; Whelan et al., 2001).

The independent variables

Demographic characteristics

Gender, aboriginal origin and interpreter needed were binary variables. The age of the individual at time of assessment was assigned to four groups: age 55–64; 65–74; 75–84; and 85 and older. Although unconventional, the age 65–74 group was assigned as the reference group because this group is experiencing many financial changes such as retirement. Marital status included four groups: married, widowed, separated or divorced and other (includes those never married or those who do not consider their status represented in any other category). Educational attainment was dichotomized at completion of grade eight as this would best represent the educational opportunities of the older cohort, especially older women. Regional divisions were at the provincial (Ontario and Nova Scotia) and regional (WRHA) level.

Health characteristics

Health characteristics were rated by the assessor using single items or a series of items comprising scales. Physical and mental health characteristics were assessed with scales that are hierarchical indices with a higher score generally reflecting greater disablement or more symptoms (Morris et al., 2000). Each scale was collapsed to a smaller group of levels as is discussed below, improving clarity for analysis and discussion (Rowe, 2006). In order to avoid arbitrary changes, guidance has come from published studies that have used summary categories.

The activities of daily living (ADL) self-performance scale (range 0 to 6) measures the disablement process in four activities: toileting, locomotion, eating and personal hygiene (Morris et al., 1999). Three levels of ADL were used in this study: independent, some impairment and functionally impaired. The instrumental activities of daily living (IADL) capacity scale measures likely difficulty with the task but not the actual performance of tasks (range 0 to 6). The three tasks are meal preparation, phone use and ordinary housework and, for this study, three levels of IADL were distinguished: no, some or great difficulty. The change in health, end-stage disease and signs and symptoms (CHESS) scale (range 0 to 5) is a strong predictor of survival and has been adapted for home care populations (Armstrong et al., 2010; Hirdes et al., 2003, 2014). For this study, CHESS scores were recoded into three levels: stable, mild, and moderate or severe instability. The cognitive performance (CPS) scale (range 0 to 6) has been validated against the Mini Mental State Examination (MMSE) (Hartmaier et al., 1995). For this study, scores were recoded into four levels: intact, mild, moderate or severe impairment. The depression rating (DRS) scale (range 0 to 14) is used to rate the mood status of the client, such as negative statements, persistent anger and signs of depression (Soldato et al., 2008). For this study, three levels of depression were distinguished: no symptoms, mild depressive symptoms or potential depression.

Dichotomous variables used in the analyses included poor self-rated health status, smoking status and number of medications (cut-off of nine to indicate polypharmacy). Psychiatric diagnosis in the past 90 days is dichotomized as "yes" for present, whether monitored or not, and "no" for not present. Whether any psychotropic medications were taken in the past seven days is also captured on the RAI-HC as a binary response.

Social support characteristics

The social support characteristics of interest in the present study are living arrangement at the time of referral, if informal helper lives with client currently, the relationships of the informal helper to the client and the number of hours of weekly informal help received. Information about living arrangements is helpful to understand the level of home care provided or required (Coyte and McKeever, 2001). Older women living alone will generally require more home care than older men living with their spouse. Sources of additional help could be informal or formal and may require out-of-pocket funding for private services or even for the travel needs of a family member (Poss et al., 2008).

Financial characteristics

The financial characteristics of interest are financial coverage by public or private insurance and the level of difficulty managing basic personal finances such as bill payments. Financial stress could increase if the client is required to pay for additional home care services due to a lack of provincial insurance coverage (insurance policy) or if financial management challenges are a possible risk to personal finances.

All data used in this study had been de-identified prior to loading into the secured database.

Analysis

Analyses were conducted using SAS software v9.2 (SAS Institute Inc., Cary, NC, USA). Initial bivariate analyses were done to identify any potential differences between those assessments missing the trade-offs value and those with completed information for the Ontario sample (n=321,817). The assessments with missing values for trade-offs (n=34,443) were dropped from further analysis.

Univariate analyses were used to fully describe the samples from all three regions as well as the overall sample with non-missing trade-off values (n=345,678). Differences between groups were tested using t-tests for continuous variables and chi-square tests for categorical variables (significance level p<0.01). Bivariate analysis for each covariate was conducted with the dependent variable "trade-offs." Odds ratios were calculated for each cross-tabulation. Predictors of risks of making economic trade-offs were identified. Variables significant at p<0.01 were retained for further multivariate analysis.

Multivariate logistic regression modeling was used to develop models for risk of economic trade-offs for the three regions combined using various selection techniques (Arunajadai, 2009; Shtatland et al., 2001). Initially, manual entry was used to test various combinations of variables based on logical groups. Variables that were found to be significant at p<0.01 and had an odds ratio outside the range of 0.75–1.50 were retained to reduce the number of covariates in the model to a reasonable size and avoid the exclusion of key variables (Shtatland et al., 2001). Some were re-entered at later stages of model testing based on information in the published literature. Ratio level variables were used both as continuous variables and as recoded nominal-level variables. Once the model was finalized by manual entry, both FORWARD and BACKWARD automatic variable selection settings were used to validate the models. Full models were run for each of the three regions following the same techniques of manual entry and validation with FORWARD and BACKWARD automatic selection that were used for the combined regions model.

Results

The total study sample size for people aged 55 and over was 380,122. The population size of the jurisdictions was: ON = 84.7 percent (n=321,817), NS = 11.6 percent (n=44,094) and WRHA = 3.7 percent (n=14,211).

Missing data analyses for the Ontario trade-offs variable were conducted. No major key demographic differences were found for those assessments with completed trade-offs (either making or not-making trade-offs) and those assessments with this variable completed inaccurately or missing. Characteristics such as mental health and frailty demonstrate some differences, but generally these types of changes are spread out over many more years than the length of this study. Those assessments missing values for trade-offs were dropped from further analysis (Shah, 2003). The final sample size was ON = 83.1 percent (n=287,374), NS = 12.8 percent (n=44,093) and WRHA = 4.1 percent (n=14,211) for a total of 345,678 assessments analyzed.

Descriptive analyses of the study population

The total study population is nearly two-thirds female and 71.1 percent (n=245,860) of the sample are age 75 or older (see Table 10.1). Most are not currently married (60.1 percent, n=207,753) but the majority have been

Table 10.1 Demographic, health and social support characteristics of each assessment region and all regions combined (n=345,678)

Variable		All subjects n=345,678 %(n)	WRHA n=14,211 %(n)	Nova Scotia n=44,093 %(n)	Ontario n=287,374 %(n)	p value
Dependent variable						
Making trade-offs	Yes	1.7 (5,982)	3.7 (532)	2.4 (1,034)	1.5 (4,416)	<0.0001
Demographics						
Aboriginal origins	Yes	0.8 (2,726)	2.1 (302)	0.1 (20)	0.8 (2,404)	<0.0001
Age (years)	55–64	11.0 (37,971)	8.8 (1,251)	11.2 (4,927)	11.1 (31,793)	<0.0001
	65–74	17.9 (61,847)	15.2 (2,159)	19.9 (8,774)	17.7 (50,914)	
	75–84	39.6 (136,924)	41.0 (5,823)	38.6 (17,004)	39.7 (114,098)	
	85+	31.5 (108,936)	35.0 (4,978)	30.4 (13,389)	31.5 (90,569)	
Education completed beyond Grade 8	Yes	76.5 (231,396)	76.2 (10,832)	n/a[a]	76.8 (220,564)	<0.0001
Gender	Female	64.4 (222,637)	69.0 (9,799)	64.5 (28,416)	64.2 (184,422)	<0.0001
Interpreter needed	Yes	20.9 (72,387)	3.4 (478)	100.0 (44,093)[a]	9.7 (27,816)	<0.0001
Marital status	Married	39.9 (137,889)	32.1 (4,568)	34.5 (15,196)	41.1 (118,125)	<0.0001
	Widowed	44.3 (153,233)	49.6 (7,054)	40.2 (17,725)	44.7 (128,454)	
	Separated/divorced	7.5 (25,832)	8.6 (1,225)	5.2 (2,279)	7.8 (22,328)	
	Other	8.3 (28,724)	9.6 (1,364)	20.2 (8,893)	6.4 (18,467)	

Variable	All subjects n=345,678 % (n)	WRHA n=14,211 % (n)	Nova Scotia n=44,093 % (n)	Ontario n=287,374 % (n)	p value
Physical health					
ADL self-performance scale					
Independent (score 0)	68.6 (236,972)	72.2 (10,253)	60.2 (26,525)	69.7 (200,194)	<0.0001
Some impairment (score 1,2)	21.2 (73,358)	19.9 (2,832)	22.1 (9,760)	21.2 (60,766)	
Functionally impaired (score 3+)	10.2 (35,346)	7.9 (1,126)	17.7 (7,808)	9.2 (26,412)	
Change in health, end-stage disease and signs and symptoms (CHESS)					
Stable (score 0)	30.3 (104,806)	35.1 (4,981)	26.0 (11,484)	30.7 (88,341)	<0.0001
Mild instability (score 1,2)	57.3 (198,006)	56.9 (8,092)	57.6 (25,391)	57.3 (164,523)	
Moderate/severe instability (score 3+)	12.4 (42,865)	8.0 (1,138)	16.4 (7,218)	12.0 (34,509)	
IADL capacity scale					
No difficulty (score 0)	6.1 (20,951)	3.1 (443)	5.7 (2,518)	6.3 (17,990)	<0.0001
Some difficulty (score 1,2,3)	25.8 (89,135)	24.1 (3,422)	19.3 (8,527)	26.9 (77,186)	
Great difficulty (score 4+)	68.2 (235,592)	72.8 (10,346)	75.0 (33,048)	66.9 (192,198)	
Poor self-rated health Yes	18.3 (63,394)	20.5 (2,917)	22.4 (9,890)	17.6 (50,587)	<0.0001
Mental health					
Cognitive Performance Scale (CPS)					
Intact (score 0)	50.6 (174,877)	54.7 (7,773)	46.5 (20,512)	51.0 (146,592)	<0.0001
Mild Impairment (score 1,2)	39.8 (137,472)	37.8 (5,369)	38.3 (16,899)	40.1 (115,204)	
Moderate Impairment (score 3,4)	6.6 (22,741)	5.6 (795)	9.6 (4,210)	6.2 (17,736)	
Severe Impairment (score 5,6)	3.1 (10,588)	1.9 (274)	5.6 (2,472)	2.7 (7,842)	

Continued

Table 10.1 *continued* Demographic, health and social support characteristics of each assessment region and all regions combined (n=345,678),

Variable		All subjects n=345,678 % (n)	WRHA n=14,211 % (n)	Nova Scotia n=44,093 % (n)	Ontario n=287,374 % (n)	p value
Depression Rating Scale (DRS)						
	None (score 0)	64.6 (223,141)	69.1 (9,813)	69.1 (30,457)	63.6 (182,871)	<0.0001
	Mild depressive symptoms (score 1,2)	22.3 (77,082)	22.3 (3,166)	21.6 (9,501)	22.4 (64,415)	
	Potential depression (score 3+)	13.2 (45,455)	8.7 (1,232)	9.4 (4,135)	14.0 (40,088)	
Psychiatric diagnosis	Yes	11.3 (38,947)	13.7 (1,943)	8.4 (3,692)	11.6 (33,312)	<0.0001
Psychiatric medications[b]	Yes	39.0 (134,684)	32.4 (4,599)	35.5 (15,649)	39.8 (114,436)	<0.0001
Health behaviors and service use						
Polypharmacy	Taking 9+ medications	43.4 (149,974)	36.0 (5,110)	34.3 (15,113)	45.1 (129,751)	<0.0001
Smoker	Yes	8.3 (28,648)	8.1 (1,145)	9.4 (4,126)	8.1 (23,377)	<0.0001
Social supports						
Informal helper lives with client	Yes	54.2 (187,204)	42.5 (6,041)	53.3 (23,480)	54.9 (157,683)	<0.0001
Informal helper weekly hours						
	0 to less than 3.5	18.9 (65,157)	24.9 (3,540)	28.8 (12,705)	17.0 (48,912)	<0.0001
	3.5 to less than 7	14.1 (48,558)	18.3 (2,607)	19.4 (8,530)	13.0 (37,421)	
	7 to less than 30	51.2 (176,882)	45.3 (6,437)	43.2 (19,044)	52.7 (151,401)	
	30+	15.9 (55,075)	11.5 (1,627)	8.7 (3,814)	17.3 (49,634)	

Variable	All subjects n=345,678 % (n)	WRHA n=14,211 % (n)	Nova Scotia n=44,093 % (n)	Ontario n=287,374 % (n)	p value
Informal helper relationship to client					
Child (in-law)	43.0 (145,293)	44.5 (6,172)	44.4 (19,580)	42.7 (119,541)	<0.0001
Spouse	31.1 (105,234)	23.8 (3,311)	24.6 (10,862)	32.5 (91,061)	
Other relative	14.6 (49,408)	19.6 (2,718)	18.3 (8,080)	13.8 (38,610)	
Friend/neighbor	11.3 (38,078)	12.1 (1,685)	12.6 (5,571)	11.0 (30,822)	
Living arrangements at referral					
Alone	36.0 (97,198)	54.6 (7,754)	42.2 (18,604)	33.4 (70,840)	<0.0001
With spouse	39.7 (107,108)	31.8 (4,514)	33.6 (14,814)	41.4 (87,780)	
With non-spouse	24.4 (65,832)	13.7 (1,943)	24.2 (10,675)	25.1 (53,214)	
Financial					
Financial management difficulty					
None (score 0)	38.5 (133,176)	41.8 (5,937)	35.5 (15,638)	38.8 (111,601)	<0.0001
Some (score 1)	25.6 (88,539)	27.1 (3,852)	22.3 (9,810)	26.1 (74,877)	
Great (score 2)	35.9 (123,962)	31.1 (4,422)	42.3 (18,645)	35.1 (100,895)	
Health insurance under provincial policy Yes	99.3 (343,138)	95.1 (13,520)	99.9 (44,074)	99.4 (285,544)	<0.0001

a Province of Nova Scotia encountered a data translation error in transmission of database and results incorrectly show 100% use of translator.
b Client is taking any one of: antipsychotic/neuroleptic, anxiolytic, antidepressant, hypnotic.

married at some point in time (91.7 percent, n=316,954) and 36.0 percent (n=97,198) currently live alone. The majority (81.7 percent, n=282,284) do not consider their health status negatively, although 8.3 percent (n=28,648) are smokers, 12.4 percent (n=42,865) are experiencing very unstable health (CHESS) and 13.2 percent (n=45,455) are showing symptoms of potential depression. Approximately one-tenth of the sample is functionally impaired (n=35,346) and moderately to severely cognitively impaired (n=33,329). During the univariate analysis, some data problems were detected in the Nova Scotia data for specific variables and they were dropped from further analysis. These variables were aboriginal origins, education and interpreter needed. Around 1.7 percent (n=5,981) of the study population made economic trade-offs, and, consequently, were experiencing poverty as defined in this study.

Univariate results in Table 10.1 comparing the total study population for each of the three regions indicate that those living in Ontario are more likely in comparison to other regions to be male, married or widowed, require an interpreter, experience more depressive symptoms, take more medications and are more positive about their health. Those in Nova Scotia are more likely to smoke, to be experiencing end-stage disease, experience higher levels of cognitive impairment and are more negative about their health. Older persons in WRHA are more likely to be making economic trade-offs, are older, female, live alone at referral, less likely to experience ADL impairments and have a psychiatric diagnosis.

Bivariate analyses were completed and the results for two covariates, health insurance under provincial policy and IADL capacity scale, were not significant at the $p < 0.01$ level and were removed from further analysis.

Multivariate analyses for making economic trade-offs

The analyses for the full model for risks of making economic trade-offs is presented in Table 10.2. All analyses used the 95 percent confidence interval. Home care clients most at risk of making trade-offs are age 55–64 (OR=2.31, 2.16–2.48), are separated or divorced (OR=2.38, 2.20–2.56), experiencing three or more depressive symptoms (OR=2.24, 2.09–2.39) and have unstable CHESS scores (OR=1.70, 1.56–1.85), smoke (OR=1.94, 1.82–2.07), have poor self-rated health (OR=1.73, 1.63–1.83) and live in the WRHA (OR=2.84, 2.58–3.13). Older age protects home care clients from making economic trade-offs. Those age 75–84 (OR=0.53, 0.49–0.56) and those age 85 or older (OR=0.32, 0.29–0.36) were less likely to be at risk of making trade-offs. Interaction effects were tested between: gender and informal caregiving hours; informal caregiver lives with client and informal caregiving hours; marital status and informal caregiver lives with client; and marital status and informal caregiving hours, but none were significant. Curvilinear effects were tested for informal caregiving hours, but were not significant.

Ontario is substantially larger than the other two regions, so its data had more influence on the results. Stratified models were run for each region to accommodate the population size differences. Table 10.2 provides the final model for each of the three regions. Two covariates, smoking and poor self-rated health, were common risks across the three regions. Reaching age 75 or older was protective in both Nova Scotia and Ontario, but not in the WRHA.

Variables significantly associated with making economic trade-offs in the bivariate analyses that did not make it into the final model were ADL impairment, CPS, psychiatric medications, polypharmacy, informal helper lives with client, informal helper weekly hours, informal helper relationship to client, living arrangements and difficulty managing finances. The final model indicates that making economic trade-offs is associated with being younger and being separated or divorced. These predictors may mean that those making trade-offs are less likely to have informal helpers available and experience less risk of experiencing ADL or CPS impairments.

Discussion

It is not entirely surprising that the youngest age group, those 55–64 years of age, was found to be at risk of making economic trade-offs since they are ineligible for most retirement and seniors' benefits. This gap in entitlements prior to age 65 can vary by province for some programs such as prescription drugs (Cheal and Kampen, 1998; Redish et al., 2006). Although some benefits are available by age 60, they are at a reduced payout level. For those aged 55–64, the combination of increased health expenses, possible decreases or loss of income due to illness plus ineligibility for most or all seniors' benefits means that many will face financial stressors, some severe enough to result in deprivation. Unfortunately, with approval of the Government of Canada 2012 budget, entitlement program policy changes planned to start in the early 2020s will gradually increase age eligibility and also increase financial risks for pre-retirement cohorts experiencing health issues.

The results from the province of Nova Scotia indicated the highest risk for the working 55–64 age group. This jurisdiction uses income means testing for residents to access home care services. Considering that this working age group is generally not eligible for seniors' benefits, they may be losing employment income as well as acquiring more health expenses than older age groups. Post-employment age seniors are more likely to have lower incomes than working age individuals, resulting in eligibility for home care benefits. The working age individual may appear to have greater means since their health issues are relatively recent. Personal income tax reporting, often used for identifying income levels, lags behind any abrupt change in income. Consequently, an unanticipated loss of income may place them into a financial crisis with no official financial evidence to demonstrate this reality. The home care health setting is especially sensitive to abrupt financial

Table 10.2 Multivariate analysis of predictors for making economic trade-offs (n=345,677)

Independent variables		All regions n=345,677 c=.79	WRHA n=14,211 c=.68	Nova Scotia n=44,093 c=.77	Ontario n=287,373 c=.78
Demographics					
Region (reference: Ontario)					
	NS	1.50 (1.40, 1.62)****			
	WRHA	2.84 (2.58, 3.13)****			
Age (years) (reference: 65–74)					
	55–64	2.31 (2.16, 2.48)****		2.96 (2.53, 3.46)****	2.25 (2.07, 2.44)****
	75–84	0.52 (0.49, 0.56)****		0.43 (0.36, 0.52)****	0.52 (0.48, 0.57)****
	85+	0.32 (0.29, 0.36)****		0.26 (0.21, 0.34)****	0.31 (0.28, 0.35)****
Marital status (reference: married)					
	Widowed	1.48 (1.38, 1.59)****			1.57 (1.45, 1.71)****
	Separated or divorced	2.38 (2.20, 2.56)****			2.52 (2.32, 2.75)****
	Other	1.85 (1.70, 2.01)****			1.90 (1.71, 2.11)****
Physical health					
Poor self-rated health	Yes	1.73 (1.63, 1.83)****	2.70 (2.25, 3.23)****	2.14 (1.88, 2.43)****	1.68 (1.57, 1.79)****
Change in health, end-stage disease and signs and symptoms (CHESS) (reference: stable, score 0)					
	Mild (score 1,2)	1.34 (1.26, 1.43)****			1.44 (1.33, 1.55)****
	Moderate/severe (score 3+)	1.70 (1.56, 1.85)****			1.85 (1.68, 2.05)****

Independent variables		All regions n=345,677 c=.79	WRHA n=14,211 c=.68	Nova Scotia n=44,093 c=.77	Ontario n=287,373 c=.78
Mental health					
Depression Rating Scale (DRS) (reference: no symptoms-score 0)					
Mild depressive symptoms (score 1,2)		1.56 (1.46, 1.65)[****]			1.50 (1.40, 1.62)[****]
Potential depression (score 3+)		2.24 (2.09, 2.39)[****]			2.27 (2.10, 2.45)[****]
Psychiatric diagnosis	Yes		1.63 (1.32, 2.01)[****]		
Health behaviors and service use					
Smoker	Yes	1.94 (1.82, 2.07)[****]	3.35 (2.70, 4.16)[****]	2.07 (1.78, 2.40)[****]	1.92 (1.79, 2.07)[****]

[****] p<0.0001.

changes because the household expenses will continue. Any policy that requires means testing will need to be sensitive to sudden income changes that can place a person at high risk of financial stress. More research on the eligibility differences for home care services between regions and client outcomes is needed.

The WRHA had the smallest and the oldest sample in the study as well as the greatest percentage of females. It was the only jurisdiction for which the modeling did not identify age as significant for making economic trade-offs. This may be because poverty in that region is more pervasive (i.e., more than double the Ontario rate) and affects even groups who are eligible for publicly funded supports. Females may be at lower risk of poverty because of their willingness to seek or accept a range of supports. They experience fewer social stigmas when encountering economic difficulties in comparison to their male counterparts and social agencies as well as families and friends may be more willing to provide support or be more aware of the need for supports.

The WRHA was also the only region for which the modeling found psychiatric diagnosis significantly associated with poverty. Mental health problems in Canadian society are stigmatized. Consequently, these individuals may face risks of poverty even in the absence of any other health risk due to barriers to earning income. A sense of a lower social status (Peretti-Watel et al., 2009; Richmond and Ross, 2008) combined with increased social exclusion provides minimal direction in helping people enter or remain in mainstream society. Home care services may be unable to meet the unique needs of the population with mental health issues. Although outside of the scope of this study, one possibility is that there is an unmet demand for psychiatric hospital beds and community mental health professionals. An inability by the region to meet this demand through mental health services results in more individuals with psychiatric diagnoses being managed through home care services where day-to-day living costs are beyond the reach of their financial means. The cross-sectional nature of the study limits the ability to better understand the length of time an individual has had a psychiatric diagnosis and if it has affected their social networks, such as living arrangements or informal caregiving hours, placing them at greater risk of poverty.

Poor self-rated health levels were significant predictors of trade-offs in each of the final models. Self-rated health scores tend to follow the rise and fall of economic levels (Brenes-Camacho, 2011; Dismuke and Egede, 2010) and the results support these findings from other studies. Smoking was also associated with poverty in all the models. This also was not surprising considering the known association between smoking and being a member of a lower socio-economic groups (Peretti-Watel et al., 2009).

Models based on both the Ontario and the total study population contained CHESS and DRS as clinical indicators as predictors of trade-offs. It is not surprising to find an association between unstable health and poverty risks. Health issues can interfere with income activities such as loss of work hours or depletion of sick leave benefits. Expenses can also increase when a health issues arises, most notably for home and personal care services such as bathing and housekeeping.

The depression variable was also a significant predictor of making trade-offs. This may suggest that the experience of depression makes it difficult to earn an income and therefore results in an increased risk of poverty. On the other hand, depression may be a response to increasing personal pressures. Self-rating of one's own health can help provide more insight on poverty risks, with the possibility of negative health perceptions accompanied by increasing need to make economic trade-offs but Ontario's results differed from the other two jurisdictions. It is interesting that even with significant CHESS (health instability) results that self-rated health had the lowest effect for Ontario clients in comparison with the other regression models. This might mean that in the absence of a severe health issue, self-rated health is influential on income, but, in Ontario's case, the reality of end-of-life issues override most of the influence of subjective health (Frijters and Ulker, 2008). It might also indicate that the cross-sectional nature of most studies does not allow an understanding of any time limit on subjective health. People come to terms with their health status, which could explain the smaller effect of poor self-rated health in Ontario clients (Gunasekara et al., 2011).

It was anticipated that for this home care population that those people who received more informal caregiving would be less likely to make trade-offs because caregivers may provide care plus other essentials such as food items. This relationship was not found to be significant. Interaction effects for informal caregiving hours were tested using gender, marital status and informal caregiver living with client but these results also were not significant. The data for informal caregiver hours from the province of Nova Scotia were understated for the year 2010 due to a data translation error at the source of data and may have reduced the overall effect of this variable in the model.

The absence of marital status as a risk factor for women was unexpected because of other research that suggests marriage protects women from poverty (Orel et al., 2004; Singh, 2006; Vignoli and De Santis, 2010). Canada has been successful in reducing poverty for seniors (MacDonald et al., 2011), with rates plummeting from 26.1 percent in 1979 to 5.2 percent in 2009 (Statistics Canada, 2011). This may explain why unmarried older women are less financially vulnerable in Canada. Canadian women are often the recipients of two inheritances: one from their parents and the other from their spouse. Widows specifically can benefit financially from asset transfers in comparison to their divorced cohorts who would be faced with asset splitting (Price and Joo, 2005). The financial fall-out from the divorce cancels any benefit from a parental inheritance. Widows, on the other hand, benefit in two ways. They are more likely to retain their family ties and this can increase social support and it can also increase financial support (Cooney and Dunne, 2001). Marital status warrants additional study because future generations of retirees will have more diverse marriage histories and longer life expectancies, potentially increasing financial challenges (Frijters and Ulker, 2008; Lin and Brown, 2012).

This study was possible across multiple regions due to the standardized assessment approach of the interRAI instruments. This not only enabled regional comparisons with very large sample sizes from diverse geographic regions in Canada but also provided a broad range of multi-disciplinary variables at an individual level. This differentiates the study from most poverty studies that have ecological data at the state or community level. The opportunity to extend this study to international populations is possible due to the standardized approach of the RAI-HC and its use in other countries and international regions. This would provide more opportunity to understand policy changes, social mores and their potential effects on populations during a time when there are increasing pressures on governments worldwide to implement austerity measures such as increasing the eligible age for entitlements

The trade-offs measure is very conservative and will not identify those who are "nearly poor" but also at high risk of making trade-offs. Poverty is not a dichotomous experience and people may be living on the cusp of poverty with diminishing well-being but are overlooked by supportive programs and policies. Risk factors identified in the final model may help with early identification of these at-risk populations who are not yet making economic trade-offs.

Although this study had a large sample size from three regions, it was drawn exclusively from home care clients and the influence of health issues on making trade-offs may not be generalizable to the Canadian adult population. The study also excluded Canadians under the age of 55 and results may be different with a younger population whose life stages are more likely to include employment income, family support and mortgage debt.

Conclusions

Although Canada provides universal healthcare insurance, not all services are recognized as essential under the Canada Health Act. Home care is deemed non-essential yet it is increasingly a preferred location of healthcare delivery for Canadians. There is no standardization of these services because policy is set by each province and territory. Individuals are faced with paying for much of this healthcare from their own pockets. Unfortunately, this places some Canadians at increased risk of poverty, morbidity and mortality. As well, those at risk are often invisible when financial measures and indicators are used that emphasise real-estate holdings and other fixed assets that provide no insight into maintenance and other financial burdens that restrict cash flow.

The multi-disciplinary nature of the interRAI assessment tool makes it possible that home care clients at risk of making detrimental economic trade-offs could be identified earlier, without monetary measures. Informal caregiving may provide one early warning method. Policy changes would be required within some jurisdictions in order to support informal caregivers and at the same time reduce client risk. Rethinking regional programs that use income cut-offs to determine eligibility for financial support or that have deductibles prior to accessing public funds is needed. These means-tested approaches, most evident in Nova Scotia, appear to be adding to the burden of residents who are not yet experiencing trade-offs but may be at risk.

The Ontario region model and the combined region full model suggest an association between economic trade-offs and health instability, depression and negative feelings about health changes. This may indicate a serious lapse in support for some of the most vulnerable in the home care population who are clinically complex and nearing the end of their lives. Those who are socially isolated due to mental health issues may be experiencing increasing financial pressures along with the burden of little or no support.

The health and social service needs of Canada's population have shifted due both to personal preference and to population aging. It appears that the national social safety net and universal healthcare programs have not yet responded to this shift, leaving provincial and territorial jurisdiction holding the proverbial "hot potato" of determining service levels and client eligibility in fiscally challenging times.

References

Armstrong, J.J., Stolee, P., Hirdes, J.P. and Poss, J.W. (2010). Examining three frailty conceptualizations in their ability to predict negative outcomes for home-care clients. *Age and Ageing*, 39, 755–758.

Arunajadai, S.G. (2009). Stepwise logistic regression. *International Anesthesia Research Society*, 109, 285.

Auger, N., Alix, C., Zang, G. and Daniel, M. (2010). Sex, age, deprivation and patterns in life expectancy in Quebec, Canada: A population-based study. *BMC Public Health*, 10, 161–169.

Brenes-Camacho, B. (2011). Favourable changes in economic well-being and self-rated health among the elderly. *Social Science & Medicine*, 72, 1228–1235.

Brown, R.L. (1991). *Economic Security in an Aging Population*. Toronto, ON: Butterworths Canada.

Bryant, T., Raphael, D., Schrecker, T. and Labonte, R. (2011). Canada: A land of missed opportunity for addressing the social determinants of health. *Health Policy*, 101, 44–58.

Butterworth, P., Rodgers, B. and Windsor, T.D. (2009). Financial hardship, socioeconomic position and depression: Results from the PATH through life survey. *Social Science & Medicine*, 69, 229–237.

Carpenter, I. and Hirdes, J.P. (2013). Using interRAI assessment systems to measure and maintain quality of long-term care. *OECD Health Policy Studies A Good Life in Old Age? Monitoring and Improving Quality in Long-term Care*, ISSN: 2074-319X (online).

Cheal, D. and Kampen, K. (1998). Poor and dependent seniors in Canada. *Ageing & Society*, 18, 147–166.

Chiriboga, D.A., Black, S.A., Aranda, M.P. and Markides, K.S. (2002). Stress and depressive symptoms among Mexican American elderly. *Journals of Gerontology, Series B: Psychological Sciences and Social Sciences*, 57, 559–568.

Cooney, T.M. and Dunne, K. (2001). Intimate relationships in later life: Current realities, future prospects. *Journal of Family Issues*, 22, 838–858.

Coyte, P.C. and McKeever, P. (2001). Home care in Canada: Passing the buck. *Canadian Journal of Nursing Research*, 33, 11–25.

Dismuke, C.E. and Egede, L.E. (2010). Association between major depression, depressive symptoms and personal income in U.S. adults with diabetes. *General Hospital Psychiatry*, 32, 484–491.

Esser, I. and Palme, J. (2010). Do public pensions matter for health and wellbeing among retired persons? Basic and income security pensions across 13 Western European countries. *International Journal of Social Welfare*, 19, S105–S120.

Frijters, P. and Ulker, A. (2008). Robustness in health research: Do differences in health measures, techniques, and time frame matter? *Journal of Health Economics*, 27, 1626–1644.

Goodridge, D., Buckley, A., Marko, J., Steeves, M., Turner, H. and Whitehead, S. (2011). Home care clients in the last year of life: Is material deprivation associated with service characteristics? *Journal of Aging and Health*, 23, 954–973.

Gray, L.C., Berg, K., Fries, B.E., Henrard, J.C., Hirdes, J.P., Steel, K. and Morris, J.N. (2009). Sharing clinical information across care settings: The birth of an integrated assessment system. *BMC Health Services Research*, 9(1), 71.

Gunasekara, F.I., Carter, K. and Blakely, T. (2011). Change in income and change in self-rated health: Systematic review of studies using repeated measures to control for confounding bias. *Social Science & Medicine*, 72, 193–201.

Hartmaier, S.L., Sloane, P.D., Guess, H.A. and Koch, G.C. (1995). Validation of the minimum data set cognitive performance scale: Agreement with the Mini-Mental State Examination. *Journals of Gerontology, Series A: Biological Sciences and Medical Sciences*, 50, M128–M133.

Haveman, R., Holden, K., Wolfe, B. and Sherlund, S. (2006). Do newly retired workers in the United States have sufficient resources to maintain well-being? *Economic Inquiry*, 44, 249–264.

Hawes, C., Fries, B.C., James, M.L. and Guihan, M. (2007). Prospects and pitfalls: Use of the RAI-HC Assessment by the Department of Veterans Affairs for home care clients. *The Gerontologist*, 47, 378–387.

Health Canada (2011). *Provincial and Territorial Home Care Programs: A Synthesis for Canada*. Retrieved from www.hc-sc.gc.ca/hcs-sss/pubs/home-domicile/1999-pt-synthes/index-eng.php#s2a4.

Hirdes, J.P. (2006). Addressing the health needs of frail elderly people: Ontario's experience with an integrated health information system. *Age and Ageing*, 35(4), 329–331.

Hirdes, J.P. and Forbes, W.F. (1989). Estimates of the relative risk of mortality based on the Ontario longitudinal study of aging. *Canadian Journal on Aging*, 8, 222–237.

Hirdes, J.P., Frijters, D.H. and Teare, G.F. (2003). The MDS-CHESS scale: A new measure to predict mortality in institutionalized older people. *Journal of the American Geriatrics Society*, 51, 96–100.

Hirdes, J.P., Ljunggren, G., Morris, J.N., Frijters, D.H.M., Finne Soveri, H., Gray, L., Bjorkgren, M. and Gilgen, R. (2008). Reliability of the interRAI suite of assessment instruments: A 12-country study of an integrated health information system. *BMC Health Services Research*, 8, 277–288.

Hirdes, J.P., Poss, J.W., Mitchell, L., Korngut, L. and Heckman, G. (2014). Use of the interRAI CHESS scale to predict mortality among persons with neurological conditions in three care settings. *PLoS One*, 9(6), e99066.

Hyde, M., Ferrie, J., Higgs, P., Heim, G. and Nazreoo, J. (2004). The effects of pre-retirement factors and retirement route on circumstances in retirement: Findings from the Whitehall II study. *Ageing & Society*, 24, 279–296.

Jariah, M., Sharifah, A.H. and Tengku Aizan, H. (2006). Perceived income adequacy and health status among older persons in Malaysia. *Asia Pacific Journal of Public Health*, 18, 2–8.

Lawton, M.P., Winter, L., Kleban, M.H. and Ruckdeschel, K. (1999). Affect and quality of life. Objective and subjective. *Journal of Aging and Health*, 11, 169–198.

Lin, I. and Brown, S.L. (2012). Unmarried boomers confront old age: A national portrait. *The Gerontologist*, 52, 153–165.

Lindeboom, M., Portrait, F. and van den Berg, G.J. (2002). An econometric analysis of the mental-health effects of major events in the life of older individuals. *Health Economics*, 11, 505–520.

Lusardi, A. and Mitchell, O.S. (2009). *How Ordinary Consumers Make Complex Economic Decisions: Financial Literacy and Retirement Readiness*. National Bureau of Economic Research. Retrieved from www.nber.org/papers/w15350.

MacDonald, B., Moore, K.D., Chen, H. and Brown, R.L. (2011). The Canadian national retirement risk index: Employing statistics Canada's lifepaths to measure the financial security of future Canadian seniors. *Canadian Public Policy*, 37, S73–S94.

Morris, J.N., Carpenter, I., Berg, K. and Jones, R.N. (2000). Outcome measures for use with home care clients. *Canadian Journal on Aging*, 19, 87–105.

Morris, J.N., Fries, B.E. and Morris, S.A. (1999). Scaling ADLs within the MDS. *Journals of Gerontology, Series A: Biological Sciences and Medical Sciences*, 54, M546–M553.

Morris, J.N., Fries, B.E., Steel, K., Ikegami, N., Bernabei, R., Carpenter, G.I., Gilgen, R., Hirdes, J.P. and Topinková, E. (1997). Comprehensive clinical assessment in community setting: Applicability of the MDS-HC. *Journal of the American Geriatrics Society*, 45(8), 1017–1024.

Nathan, H. and Pawlik, T.M. (2007). Limitations of claims and registry data in surgical oncology research. *Annals of Surgical Oncology*, 15, 415–425.

Nolan, B. and Whelan, C.T. (2010). Using non-monetary deprivation indicators to analyze poverty and social exclusion: Lessons from Europe. *Journal of Policy Analysis and Management*, 29, 305–325.

Orel, N.A., Ford, R.A. and Brock, C. (2004). Women's financial planning for retirement: The impact of disruptive life events. *Journal of Women & Aging*, 16, 39–53.

Peretti-Watel, P., Seror, V., Constance, J. and Beck, F. (2009). Poverty as a smoking trap. *International Journal of Drug Policy*, 20, 230–236.

Poss, J.W., Hirdes, J.P., Fries, B.E., McKillop, I. and Chase, M. (2008). Validation of resource utilization groups version III for home care (RUG-III/HC): Evidence from a Canadian home care jurisdiction. *Medical Care*, 46, 380–387.

Price, C.A. and Joo, E. (2005). Exploring the relationship between marital status and women's retirement satisfaction. *International Journal of Aging and Human Development*, 61, 37–55.

Raghunathan, T.E. (2004). What do we do with missing data? Some options for analysis of incomplete data. *Annual Review of Public Health*, 25, 99–117.

Raphael, D. (2002). Poverty, income inequality and health in Canada. Ontario: CSJ Foundation for Research and Education. Retrieved from www.povertyandhumanrights.org/docs/incomeHealth.pdf.

Raphael, D. (2007). *Poverty and Policy in Canada: Implications for Health and Quality of Life*. Toronto: Canadian Scholars' Press.

Rappaport, A.M. and Siegel, S. (2009). Financial literacy and the challenges of the postretirement period. *Benefits Quarterly*, 25(3), 7–10.

Redish, A., Sarra, J. and Schabas, M. (2006). Growing old gracefully: An investigation into the growing number of bankrupt Canadians over age 55. Funded by Office of the Superintendent of Bankruptcy, March 21.

Richmond, C.A.M. and Ross, N.A. (2008). Social support, material circumstance and health behavior: Influences on health in First Nation and Inuit communities of Canada. *Social Science & Medicine*, 67, 1423–1433.

Ross, D.P., Scott, K.J. and Smith, P.J. (2000). *The Canadian Fact Book on Poverty 2000*. Ottawa: Canadian Council on Social Development.

Rowe, K. (2006). The measurement of composite variables from multiple indicators: Applications in quality assurance and accreditation systems—childcare. Background paper for National Childcare Accreditation Council. Retrieved from http://ncac.acecqa.gov.au/reports/report-documents/composite_variables.pdf.

Sachs-Erricsson, N., Corsentino, E. and Cougle, J.R. (2009). Problems meeting basic needs predict cognitive decline in community-dwelling Hispanic older adults. *Journal of Aging and Health*, 21, 848–863.

Saunders, P. and Adelman, L. (2006). Income poverty, deprivation and exclusion: A comparative study of Australia and Britain. *Journal of Social Policy*, 35, 559–584.

Shah, B.V. (2003). Hosmer-Lemeshow goodness of fit test for survey data. *2003 Joint Statistical Meeting*—section on survey Research Methods, pp. 3778–3781.

Sharratt, A. (2015). "I didn't die." Cancer free with no retirement savings. *The Globe and Mail*, November 21. Retrieved from www.theglobeandmail.com/globe-investor/retirement/retire-health/preparing-for-the-cost-of-catastrophic-illnesses-before-retirement/article27325454.

Shtatland, E.S., Cain, E. and Barton, M.B. (2001). The perils of stepwise logistic regression and how to escape them using information criteria and the output delivery system. *SAS User Group Paper 222–26*. Retrieved from http://www2.sas.com/proceedings/sugi26/p222-26.pdf.

Singh, S. (2006). Perceived health among women retirees. *Psychological Studies*, April–June, 166–170.

Soldato, M., Liperoti, R., Landi, F., Carpenter, I.G., Bernabei, R. and Onder, G. (2008). Patient depression and caregiver attitudes: Results from the aged in home care study. *Journal of Affective Disorders*, 106, 107–115.

Statistics Canada (2011). *Income in Canada 2009*. (Tables 202–0802 and 202–0804). Ottawa: Statistics Canada (Catalogue No. 75-202-X).

Szanton, S.L., Allen, J.K., Thorpe, R.J. Jr., Seeman, T., Bandeen-Roche, K. and Fried, L.P. (2008). Effect of financial strain on mortality in community-dwelling older women. *Journals of Gerontology, Series B: Psychological Sciences and Social Sciences*, 63, S369–S374.

Szanton, S.L., Thorpe, R.J. and Whitfield, K. (2010). Life-course financial strain and health in African-Americans. *Social Science & Medicine*, 71, 259–265.

Vignoli, D. and De Santis, G. (2010). Individual and contextual correlates of economic difficulties in old age in Europe. *Population Research and Policy Review*, 29, 481–501.

Whelan, C.T., Layte, R., Maître, B. and Nolan, B. (2001). Income, deprivation and economic strain: An analysis of the European community household panel. *European Sociological Review*, 17, 357–372.

Williamson, D.L. (2000). Health behaviours and health: Evidence that the relationship is not conditional on income adequacy. *Social Science & Medicine*, 51, 1741–1754.

11 Do fuzzy retirement-income systems work best?

Brian K. Gran

Across the globe, experts decry long-term prospects of public pension systems. Public pensions will run out of cash before they meet commitments. Public pensions are too expensive; governments cannot afford to pay them (see Barr, 2006 for an excellent overview). Global competition prevents governments from raising taxes, leaving public pension programs on paths to inadequacy, if not insolvency (Schwartz, 2001).

Yet private pensions are vulnerable to vagaries of financial markets. Private pensions can shrink when the stock market declines. Employers can and do offer narrower commitments to their employees' retirement security when unemployment is high and chronic. What can a person do? If the answer is to save, this solution is difficult to achieve when wages are stagnant and household and personal expenses are on the rise (Ebbinghaus and Wiß, 2010; Rowlingson, 2002).

A response found across various societies is fuzzy public–private retirement-income systems. In these systems, multi-faceted approaches are employed to produce retirement-income security. Do these fuzzy public–private retirement-income systems succeed in promoting economic security? Closely examining contemporary evidence of retirement-income security of thirty-four OECD countries, this chapter investigates whether public–private options succeed in achieving retirement-income security. We find that retirement-income security arises from select configurations of public–private pensions, as well as other factors, such as a society's system of taxes and transfers.

Background

The seminal work of Asa Briggs in 1961 defined the welfare state as consisting of three components:

> A "welfare state" is a state in which organized power is deliberately used (through politics and administration) in an effort to modify the play of market forces in at least three directions—first, by guaranteeing individuals and families a minimum income irrespective of the

market value of their work or their property; second, by narrowing the extent of insecurity by enabling individuals and families to meet certain "social contingencies" (for example, sickness, old age and unemployment) which lead otherwise to individual and family crises; and third, by ensuring that all citizens without distinction of status or class are offered the best standards available in relation to a certain agreed range of social services.

(Briggs, 1961, p. 228)

These three components seem designed to achieve three distinct purposes. The first purpose is to guarantee a minimum income to all individuals and families. The second purpose is to protect all individuals and families from crises and predictable events, such as older age. The third purpose is to provide highest quality of social services to citizens, as opposed to all individuals and families. Few contemporary welfare states take all three approaches. Instead, most rely on one or two approaches. In the case of retirement pensions, some societies employ the first of Briggs' approaches, guaranteeing minimum incomes, or the second, insurance against unemployment during retirement. Some societies employ a hybrid of Briggs' first and second approaches. Before we investigate contemporary approaches to retirement-income security, let's place public pensions in a historical perspective.

Retirement pensions became a welfare state responsibility in Germany in 1889 (Börsch-Supan and Schnabel, 1998), in Denmark in 1891 (Overbye, 1997) and in New Zealand in 1898 (St. John and Gran, 2001). These public pension programs were distinct in their approaches. Germany provided contribution-based pensions to industrial workers, by which workers, employers and the state contributed to the pension plan (Overbye, 1997; cf. Hinrichs and Kangas, 2003). Denmark and New Zealand, in contrast, made available to all citizens means-tested pensions that were tax financed (Overbye, 1997). These two approaches fit Briggs' first (Denmark and New Zealand) and second (Germany) approaches to providing welfare. Since the establishment of the German, Danish and New Zealand approaches, not only have national governments of these countries reformed their public pension programs, countries across the world now offer public pension programs of different shapes and sizes.

Since Briggs' groundbreaking work, a significant move forward in welfare state scholarship is Gøsta Esping-Andersen's (1990, 1999) *The Three Worlds of Welfare Capitalism* and *Social Foundations of Postindustrial Societies*. In contrast to Briggs' notion of the welfare state, Esping-Andersen put forth the concept of *welfare regimes*. A welfare regime consists of efforts of individuals, households and families, and market actors, including employers (Esping-Andersen, 1999). Private pensions are a component of Esping-Andersen's regime idea. The three worlds Esping-Andersen (1990, 1999) identified are social democratic, conservative and liberal. A social democratic welfare regime primarily provides retirement-income security through public pensions, with an emphasis on redistribution. A conservative welfare regime also provides retirement-income security through public pensions, but its emphasis is on maintaining social status of families. A liberal welfare regime primarily provides retirement-income security through the market, with an emphasis on placing risk on individuals.

Since publication of *The Three Worlds* and *Social Foundations*, scholars have studied politics of private welfare states (Hacker, 2002), configurations of public–private social policies (Gran, 2003) and how parties and institutions shape public and private welfare programs (Béland and Gran, 2008; Pierson, 2001). This scholarship influenced and was influenced by debates over dilemmas facing public pension programs.

As we know, experts claim that public pension systems are on the verge of collapse. In fact, experts have claimed that public pension systems have been on the verge of collapse for twenty years or so. In *Averting the Old Age Crisis*, World Bank (1994) experts raised alarms about aging populations and their consequences, including bankruptcy of public pension plans. To put it succinctly, World Bank experts feared too many older people would need public pensions, that older individuals had inadequately saved for retirement and public pension plans were not properly designed to pay pensions to a large group of people who live long lives.

In response to the concerns of the World Bank and others, governments turned to private pensions as a way to avert the old age crisis. Considering OECD countries, private pension assets have increased since 2008 (OECD, 2015a; Turner and Rajnes, 2014). In the ten-year period from 2004 to 2014, total assets in pension funds of OECD countries increased from $14.8 trillion in 2004 to $25.2 trillion in 2014. It is important to note that total assets in pension funds of OECD countries dropped from $1.7 trillion in a single year, from $19.5 trillion in 2007 to $17.8 trillion in 2008 (OECD, 2015a).

Quickly, evidence piled up that complete reliance on private pensions was not the answer. Indeed, complete reliance could be dangerous. First heralded as a shining example, the Chilean approach to private pensions led to crisis (Rohter, 2006). The Chilean approach was mandating individuals to contribute to personal accounts. One weakness was coverage was inadequate. Another weakness was costs, particularly costs companies charged to manage the individual accounts.

Some experts recommended that public–private mixes of pension plans were a better answer. A private pension plan, for instance, could complement a public pension plan. One example is found in the recommendations made by US President George W. Bush's Commission to Strengthen Social Security (2001), which recommended three alternatives, all three of which incorporated personal voluntary accounts. This report failed to gain traction, one reason being its length—256 pages. Another reason is what happened on September 11, 2001, in the United States. US citizens and residents, as well as their leaders, turned their attention to more immediate concerns, rather than this report, published in December 2001. Later President George W. Bush tried to persuade US citizens and residents to pay attention to the "blue ribbon report," but lack of interest in the report's findings and recommendations resulted in the report's placement in the policy trash bin.

As experts early on pointed out, there are varieties of public–private mixes to consider. This chapter examines public–private mixes found in OECD member countries. It will take a close look at contemporary configurations of retirement pensions, then explore which systems provide retirement-income security. Which do "best" when it comes to providing retirement-income security?

For purposes of this study, the OECD (2015b) characterizes the first tier of public pensions as one of three types: targeted, basic and minimum. A targeted plan is intended to provide a benefit to older individuals whose incomes are low. A basic plan either provides the same benefit to every older individual or is designed to reflect years of work, but not earnings. Receipt of the basic plan is not affected by other income, including other pensions. Whether or not an individual has income from other pensions, a minimum pension ensures that an individual enjoys a specified income during retirement (OECD, 2015b). The OECD's (2015b) second tier includes a public, employment-based pension and public, defined-contribution pension, as well as two private pensions, a defined-contribution and a defined-benefit plan. A defined-contribution plan is when the plan's sponsor is obligated to make a defined contribution, but not obligated to ensure a resulting balance. The risk of ensuring a sufficient balance lies on the future retiree. A defined-benefit plan, on the other hand, is when the plan's sponsor guarantees a resulting balance. The risk of ensuring a sufficient balance lies on the plan's sponsor (OECD Working Party on Private Pensions, 2005). Of the thirty-four OECD members this chapter examines, it is important to note that none uses a public defined-contribution approach.

Time period and case selection

For purposes of this chapter, we focus on contemporary provision of retirement pensions. For the retirement-income systems we study, we examine the year 2013, with the exception of Canada, for which evidence is from 2011, and the United Kingdom, for which evidence is from 2012. We examine Gini coefficients and poverty levels for the year 2013.

This study concentrates on public and private pension programs in thirty-four countries. These countries are OECD members found in Asia, Europe, North America and Oceania, plus Chile, the first South American OECD member. An advantage of this chapter is Chile's inclusion given its experiments with private pension plans.

Analysis

Public and private efforts

Dividing the retirement pension world into public and private, we observe stark contrasts among the thirty-four countries' approaches to retirement pensions (Table 11.1). The focus is on what the OECD calls the first and second tiers.

Table 11.1 Public and private efforts to provide retirement income in first and second tiers

Country	Public	Private
Australia	38.8	61.2
Austria	100	0
Belgium	100	0
Canada (2011)	100	0
Chile	17	83
Czech Republic	100	0
Denmark	45.2	54.8
Estonia	57.6	42.4
Finland	100	0
France	100	0
Germany	100	0
Greece	100	0
Hungary	100	0
Iceland	14.8	85.2
Ireland	100	0
Israel	34	66
Italy	100	0
Japan	100	0
Korea	100	0
Luxembourg	100	0
Mexico	27.5	72.5
The Netherlands	36.7	63.3
New Zealand	100	0
Norway	88.8	11.2
Poland	51.1	48.9
Portugal	100	0
Slovak Republic	57.8	42.2
Slovenia	100	0
Spain	100	0
Sweden	55.6	44.4
Switzerland	65.4	34.6
Turkey	100	0
United Kingdom (2012)	100	0
United States	100	0

Source: OECD (2015b).

Considering the first and second tiers of these thirty-four countries' retirement-income systems, we observe noticeable differences. Of the OECD members, twenty-one exclusively rely on public programs to provide retirement income as part of their first and second tiers.

Private pension plans are part of second-tier efforts to provide retirement-income security for thirteen OECD members. For seven of the OECD members, over 50 percent of first and second tiers arise from private pensions. The same is true for another four members, for which private pension plans account for 40 percent.

Kinds of public and private efforts

We investigate which retirement-income systems rely on types of public pensions in their first and second tiers of retirement-income security.[1] The first tier is designed to ensure that older individuals enjoy a modicum of living standards (Esping-Andersen, 1990). The second tier is designed to ensure that older individuals enjoy a standard of living comparable to when they were working. According to the OECD's approach, both the first and second tiers are mandatory, although a person living in a country where all approaches are available will not necessarily receive income from all components (OECD, 2013).

We examine approaches by type, starting with an examination of countries whose pension systems include a public, *targeted* pension (Table 11.2). This group is composed of Australia (38.8 percent), Canada (17.8 percent), Chile (17 percent), Denmark (19.8 percent), Iceland (2.9 percent), Slovenia (6.3 percent) and the United Kingdom (0.1 percent). Of these plans, Australia, Chile and Slovenia only use targeted plans as their first tier. They do not use basic or minimum plans. On the other hand, Canada, Denmark, Iceland and the United Kingdom employ an additional type of first-tier pension, with Canada, Denmark and Iceland using basic pensions, as well.

Retirement-income systems of some countries rely on *basic* pensions to provide first-tier retirement income (Table 11.2). The Czech Republic (18.2 percent), Estonia (29.4 percent), Ireland (100 percent), Israel (34 percent), Japan (42.7 percent), Korea (54.1 percent), the Netherlands (36.7 percent) and New Zealand (100 percent) only employ a basic pension as their first tier. The basic pension is the only pension of the first and second tiers of Ireland and New Zealand. For the other retirement-income systems that only use basic pensions as the first tier, three systems only use employment-related pensions as the second tier: the Czech Republic (81.8 percent), Japan (42.7 percent) and Korea (45.9 percent).

Of the countries whose retirement-income systems employ *minimum* pensions as their first tier, only Greece, Mexico and the United Kingdom significantly employ minimum pensions, with Greece at 45 percent, Mexico at 15.6 percent and the United Kingdom at 36.4 percent. Of the other retirement-income systems that employ minimum pensions, some minimum

Table 11.2 Types of public and private pensions

Country	Public: targeted	Public: basic	Public: minimum	Public: employment related	Private: defined benefit	Private: defined contribution
Australia	38.8	0	0	0	0	61.2
Austria	0	0	0	100	0	0
Belgium	0	0	2.1	97.9	0	0
Canada (2011)	17.8	31.7	0	50.5	0	0
Chile	17	0	0	0	0	83
Czech Republic	0	18.2	0	81.8	0	0
Denmark	19.8	25.4	0	0	0	54.8
Estonia	0	29.4	0	28.2	0	42.4
Finland	0	0	0.5	99.5	0	0
France	0	0	0	100	0	0
Germany	0	0	0	100	0	0
Greece	0	0	45	55	0	0
Hungary	0	0	0	0	0	0
Iceland	2.9	11.9	0	0	85.2	0
Ireland	0	100	0	0	0	0
Israel	0	34	0	0	0	66
Italy	0	0	0	100	0	0
Japan	0	42.7	0	57.3	0	0
Korea	0	54.1	0	45.9	0	0
Luxembourg	0	20.2	1.9	77.9	0	0
Mexico	0	11.9	15.6	0	0	72.5
The Netherlands	0	36.7	0	0	63.3	0
New Zealand	0	100	0	0	0	0
Norway	0	0	0.7	88.1	0	11.2
Poland	0	0	0	51.1	0	48.9
Portugal	0	0	2.8	97.2	0	0
Slovak Republic	0	0	0	57.8	0	42.2
Slovenia	6.3	0	0	93.7	0	0
Spain	0	0	0	100	0	0
Sweden	0	0	3.1	52.5	0	44.4
Switzerland	0	0	0	65.4	34.6	0
Turkey	0	0	1.1	98.9	0	0
United Kingdom (2012)	0.1	51	36.4	12.5	0	0
United States	0	0	0	100	0	0

Source: OECD (2015b).

pensions only contribute modest amounts to average pension wealth, ranging from 0.5 percent and 0.7 percent (Finland and Norway, respectively) to 1.1 percent and 2.1 percent (Turkey and Belgium, respectively) to 2.8 percent and 3.1 percent (Portugal and Sweden, respectively). For those countries that exclusively rely on minimum pensions as their first tier and yet their minimum pension only provides a modest level of wealth, their retirement-income systems' second tiers all use public employment-related pensions, with Belgium at 97.9 percent, Finland at 99.5 percent, Norway at 88.1 percent, Portugal at 97.2 percent, Sweden at 52.5 percent and Turkey at 98.9 percent.

Retirement-income systems of some countries solely utilize *employment-related* pensions, all of which are second-tier sources. These retirement-income systems do not employ first-tier components. These retirement-income systems include Austria (100 percent), France (100 percent), Germany (100 percent), Hungary (100 percent), Italy (100 percent), Spain (100 percent) and the United States (100 percent). Other retirement-systems do not exclusively use employment-related pensions, but to a large degree do rely on employment-related pensions, such as Belgium at 97.9 percent, Finland at 99.5 percent, Portugal at 97.2 percent and Turkey at 98.9 percent.

The public retirement pension plans of some countries are more complicated. According to the OECD, Canada's public pension plan consists of two first-tier components and one second-tier component. The first tier consists of a targeted pension and a basic pension. On average, the targeted pension provides 17.8 percent and the basic pension provides 31.7 percent to average pension wealth. Canada's second tier consists of a public earnings-related pension, which provides 50.5 percent to average pension wealth. Canada is not alone. Similar approaches are taken by the retirement-income systems of Denmark, Iceland, Luxembourg, Mexico and the United Kingdom. The retirement-income systems of Denmark and Iceland employ targeted and basic pensions as their first tiers, then private pensions as their second tiers. Norway and Sweden's retirement-income systems rely on minimum pensions as their first tier, then public employment-related pensions and private, defined-contribution plans as their second tiers. Luxembourg's retirement-income system employs targeted and minimum pensions as its first tier, then public, employment-related pension as its second tier. Mexico's retirement-income system takes a similar approach to Luxembourg's first tier, but its second tier relies on private, defined-contribution pensions.

Retirement-income security? Inequality

Given that many of the retirement-income systems of the examined countries emphasize public efforts, may we expect greater income security among individuals who are age 65 and older? We examine two characteristics of groups of people age 65 and older across these thirty-four countries, inequality and poverty. For each analysis, we examine a "before" and "after" indicator (Table 11.3). One of our primary questions is whether countries that rely on public pensions are associated with less inequality and lower poverty levels. Another question is whether one type of public pension, or a combination of public pensions, is associated with lower inequality and poverty levels.

Table 11.3 Inequality among individuals who are age 65 or older for 2012

Country	Gini of gross income before taxes	Gini of disposable income post taxes and transfers	Gini reduction
Australia	.705	.316	0.389
Austria	.874	.268	0.606
Belgium	.929	.229	0.7
Canada (2011)	.548	.274	0.274
Chile (2011)	.528	.465	0.063
Czech Republic	.859	.199	0.66
Denmark	.636	.214	0.422
Estonia	.811	.256	0.555
Finland	.868	.252	0.616
France	.784	.3	0.484
Germany	.765	.269	0.496
Greece	.895	.267	0.628
Hungary	.763	.225	0.538
Iceland	.738	.242	0.496
Ireland	.879	.29	0.589
Israel	.608	.382	0.226
Italy	.801	.298	0.503
Japan (2009)	.694	.341	0.353
Korea	.531	.43	0.101
Luxembourg	.882	.28	0.602
Mexico	.553	.512	0.041
The Netherlands	.54	.232	0.308
New Zealand	.647	.311	0.336
Norway	.588	.216	0.372
Poland	.777	.249	0.528
Portugal	.826	.328	0.498
Slovak Republic	.772	.195	0.577
Slovenia	.842	.257	0.585
Spain	.745	.292	0.453
Sweden	.619	.277	0.342
Switzerland	.539	.297	0.242
Turkey	.466	.379	0.087
United Kingdom	.336	.316	0.02
United States	.712	.401	0.311

Source: OECD (2015c).

For purposes of this study, inequality is measured as a Gini coefficient. The Gini coefficient is frequently used to indicate income inequality (UNDP 2015; World Bank, 2015; but see Atkinson and Morelli, 2014). One reason the Gini coefficient is attractive is that it is a single number. This number ranges from 0, perfect equality, to 1, perfect inequality. For this study, we focus on inequality among individuals who are age 65 and older. We examine Gini coefficients for 2012, except the indicators for Canada and Chile are from 2011 and for Japan they are from 2009 (OECD, 2015c).

What can we say about the relationship between retirement-income systems and inequality? In a word, a public emphasis does not necessarily lead to low levels of inequality. Let's take a closer look.

Among those countries with high Gini scores (>.3) post taxes and transfers, i.e., Australia, France, Israel, Japan, Korea, Mexico, New Zealand, Portugal, Turkey, the United Kingdom and the United States, some of these countries are characterized as distributing 100 percent of first- and second-tier pension wealth through public programs. That is, according to the OECD, the first and second tiers of their retirement-income systems do not turn to private pensions. This subset of countries includes France, Japan, Korea, New Zealand, Portugal, Turkey, the United Kingdom and the United States. Despite their use of public pensions in the first and second tiers, older individuals living in these countries experience high inequality.

Among those countries with high Gini scores (>.3) post taxes and transfers, incorporation of private pensions into the second tier (not one uses private in primary) does not automatically lead to high inequality levels during retirement. Which countries are associated with high levels of inequality?

Of those countries that employ private pensions in their second tier approaches, inequality levels are lower (<.3) among older individuals for Denmark, Estonia, the Netherlands, Norway, Poland, Slovak Republic, Sweden and Switzerland. The incorporation of private pensions in the first two tiers of retirement-income security does not automatically lead to greater inequality among older individuals.

Perhaps the incorporation of private pensions in the second tier of retirement-income security is associated with less inequality reduction. A comparison of before, a Gini of gross income before taxes, with after, a Gini of disposable income after taxes and transfers, suggests important differences in inequality reduction. Of those countries that incorporate private pensions in the first two tiers, inequality reduction is less (<.3) in Israel (.226), Mexico (.041) and Switzerland (.242). Some countries whose second tiers incorporate private approaches do manage to produce more significant reductions, including Australia (.389), Denmark (.422), Estonia (.555), the Netherlands (.308), Norway (.372), Poland (.528), the Slovak Republic (.577) and Sweden (.599).

Is reliance on public efforts in the first and second tiers strongly related to greater reductions in inequality? The clear answer is no. Of those countries with public-oriented first and second tiers, inequality reduction is less (<.3) for Canada, Korea, Turkey and the United Kingdom. One explanation of this weak inequality reduction is that the starting point was low inequality among older individuals before taxes and transfers. This explanation characterizes the United Kingdom, for which the Gini coefficient of gross income *before* taxes was lower than six countries *after* taxes and transfers, i.e., Israel, Japan, Korea, Mexico, Turkey and the United States. Another reason is that the public approaches to the first and second tiers of retirement income do not excel in providing retirement-income security.

Retirement-income security: poverty

Prevention and elimination of poverty among older individuals is often considered a goal of providing retirement income (Ghilarducci, 2007). Even if some of the public and private approaches do not reduce large proportions of inequality, are these approaches associated with low levels of poverty and high levels of poverty reduction?

We may expect that countries whose second tiers incorporate private approaches would do worse in preventing poverty and eliminating poverty. Let's investigate OECD evidence (Table 11.4). The OECD measures poverty as 50 percent of a country's median income (Keeley, 2014). This measure is one way to measure relative poverty, by which we can evaluate distribution of income across a country's population.

The poverty rate after taxes and transfers remains high for some of the countries whose second tiers include private approaches (OECD, 2015d). Australia's poverty rate among older individuals is .335, Israel's is .207, Mexico's is .27 and Switzerland's is .234. From 20 percent to over 33 percent of these countries' older individuals live at 50 percent of their countries' median income. This level of poverty among older individuals reveals that these societies permit over one-in-five, for Israel up to one-in-three, of older individuals to live in poverty.

Conversely, incorporating a private approach does not necessarily lead to high poverty levels. Poverty rates are comparatively low for Denmark, Estonia, the Netherlands, Norway, Poland, the Slovak Republic and Sweden, with less than 5 percent of older individuals living in Denmark, the Netherlands, Norway and the Slovak Republic experiencing income poverty.

Given these findings about private efforts, it may come as a surprise that relying on public pensions in first and second tiers does not necessarily prevent poverty among older individuals. Concentrating on those countries that rely on public efforts in the first two tiers of retirement income, retirement-income systems of two countries fail to prevent large proportions of their older populations from entering poverty, with the United States failing 21 percent of its older population and Korea failing an astounding 48.5 percent of its older adults.

Is a reliance on public efforts at the first and second tiers associated with greater poverty reduction? The answer is yes for the countries that rely on public efforts, with all but Korea and Turkey producing large reductions (>.4) in poverty. Of these countries whose first and second tiers rely on public efforts, many are associated with poverty reductions of .7 or higher, including Austria, Belgium, the Czech Republic, Finland, France, Germany, Greece, Hungary, Ireland, Luxembourg and Portugal.

Table 11.4 Poverty among individuals who are age 65 or older for 2012

Country	Poverty rate before taxes and transfers	Poverty rate after taxes and transfers	Poverty reduction
Australia	.678	.335	0.343
Austria	.851	.114	0.737
Belgium	.896	.107	0.789
Canada (2011)	.506	.067	0.439
Chile	.421	.205	0.216
Czech Republic	.848	.028	0.82
Denmark	.631	.046	0.585
Estonia	.808	.121	0.687
Finland	.892	.093	0.799
France	.83	.038	0.792
Germany	.818	.094	0.724
Greece	.816	.069	0.747
Hungary	.777	.056	0.721
Iceland	.731	.028	0.703
Ireland	.859	.069	0.79
Israel	.449	.207	0.242
Italy	.778	.094	0.684
Japan (2009)	.642	.194	0.448
Korea	.597	.485	0.112
Luxembourg	.811	.03	0.781
Mexico	.338	.27	0.068
The Netherlands	.621	.015	0.606
New Zealand	.588	.082	0.506
Norway	.681	.041	0.64
Poland	.725	.082	0.643
Portugal	.796	.081	0.715
Slovak Republic	.773	.036	0.737
Slovenia	.85	.158	0.692
Spain	.742	.067	0.675
Sweden	.692	.093	0.599
Switzerland	.533	.234	0.299
Turkey (2012)	.283	.172	0.111
United Kingdom (2012)	.613	.134	0.479
United States (2012)	.618	.21	0.408

Source: OECD (2015d).

Discussion and conclusion

Do fuzzy public–private retirement-income systems succeed in promoting economic security? The answer to this question is, "it depends." This chapter presents evidence that some public pension plans do promote retirement-income security, yet some public–private systems do succeed in promoting retirement-income security as well. How can this be? One part of the explanation is that the configuration of the retirement-income system seems to matter. Another part of the explanation is that the retirement-income system is a component of a socio-economic structure that shapes retirement-income security.

Can we identify types of retirement-income systems that provide security? What we can identify is multiple approaches to providing retirement-income security, as well as approaches *not* to take to provide retirement-income security.

First, if a society wants to prevent high inequality and high poverty levels among its older populations, those societies should not take the approaches of Chile, Korea, Mexico and the United States. Considering their Gini coefficients for older individuals, Chile (.465), Korea (.43), Mexico (.512) and the United States (.401) do lousy jobs in reducing inequality. Chile (.205), Korea (.485), Mexico (.27) and the United States (.21) also do lousy jobs in preventing poverty.

What do the retirement-income systems of Chile, Korea, Mexico and the United States have in common? On the face of it, little. A closer look, however, reveals that both Korea and the United States primarily rely on public earnings-related pensions, which replicate success or failure in the paid workplace. Chile and Mexico's reliance on defined contribution plans may produce a similar effect of replicating success or failure in the paid workplace.

Yet this picture only is part of the story. The other part of the story is that Chile, Korea, Mexico and the United States do not effectively use their tax systems to reduce inequality and poverty among older individuals. This combination of replicating earnings in retirement income with weak tax redistribution to a large degree explains why the Korean, Mexican and US systems do not promote retirement-income security. If providing retirement-income security is an important objective, government leaders should not take the paths pension officials of Chile, Korea, Mexico and the United States have taken.

Experts characterize private approaches as less progressive in the distribution of resources (Center on Budget Policy and Priorities, 2015). Are inequality and poverty levels higher in countries that employ private approaches to a larger degree? Considering the thirty-four OECD members studied in this chapter, the answer to this question is a resounding "maybe." While many retirement-income systems that emphasize a private approach do not promote retirement-income security, some retirement-income systems that primarily employ private approaches do succeed in promoting retirement-income security. Denmark, Iceland and the Netherlands on average provide most retirement income through either private defined-benefit or defined-contribution approaches. The retirement-income systems of Iceland (85.2 percent) and the Netherlands (63.3 percent) employ defined-benefit approaches, while Denmark's (54.8 percent) primarily employs defined-contribution approaches. Yet Denmark, Iceland and the Netherlands maintain low poverty levels (ranging from .015 to .046) and low inequality levels (from .214 to .242), among the most superior retirement-income achievements of all examined countries. How can these three countries employ private approaches while ensuring retirement-income security?

The answer to this question consists of two parts. One part is that the retirement-income systems of these countries combine public and private approaches to providing retirement income. The second part is that all three have moderately high levels of poverty, compared to their peers, *prior* to redistribution. All three also have moderately high levels of inequality *prior* to redistribution. Through taxes and transfers, including public pensions, these retirement-income systems reduce poverty and inequality, thereby providing retirement security.

While some public-oriented retirement-income systems fail to achieve retirement security, the public approaches of Belgium, the Czech Republic and Hungary are associated with low levels of poverty and inequality. What do these retirement-income systems have in common? All three use public, employment-based pensions to a large degree. On the face of it, this success in providing retirement-income security on the shoulders of employment-based pensions is a puzzle. Employment-based pensions tend to reproduce inequalities arising from the paid labor market. The answer to the puzzle seems to be that the tax and transfer systems of Belgium, the Czech Republic and Hungary significantly reduce inequality and poverty. This result suggests that taxes and transfers working in conjunction with public pension systems may lead to retirement-income security among older individuals.

Clearly one size does not fit all when it comes to retirement-income security. The answer to whether fuzzy public–private retirement-income systems succeed in promoting economic security is, it depends. Whether public and private pension plans provide retirement-income security not only depends on configurations of public and private pensions, but other factors as well, such as taxes and transfers. In sum, retirement-income security arises from a retirement-income system that not only relies on pensions, but incorporates tax and transfers.

Note

1 Omitted from this analysis are what the OECD considers to be third-tier retirement pensions. These income sources are voluntary. Governments of these OECD countries do not require their provision.

References

Atkinson, A. and Morelli, S. (2014). *The Chartbook of Economic Inequality.* Accessed December 31, 2015: www.voxeu.org/article/chartbook-economic-inequality.

Barr, N. (2006). Pensions: An overview of the issues. *Oxford Review of Economic Policy,* 22(1), 1–14.

Béland, D. and Gran, B.K. (2008). *Public and Private Social Policy*. Hampshire: Palgrave Macmillan.

Börsch-Supan, A. and Schnabel, R. (1998). Social security and declining labor-force participation in Germany. *American Economic Review*, 88(2), 173–178.

Briggs, A. (1961). The welfare state in historical perspective. *Archives Europeennes de Sociologie, II*, 221–258. Accessed: www.econ.boun.edu.tr/content/2015/summer/EC-48B01/Lecture%20Note-3_Briggs_2006-06-29-2015.pdf.

Center on Budget and Policy Priorities (2015). *Policy Basics: Top Ten Facts about Social Security*. Accessed December 31, 2015: www.cbpp.org/research/social-security/policy-basics-top-ten-facts-about-social-security.

Ebbinghaus, B. and Wiß, T. (2010). The governance and regulation of private pensions in Europe. In Bernard Ebbinghaus (ed), *The Varieties of Pension Governance* (pp. 351–383). Oxford: Oxford University Press.

Esping-Andersen, G. (1990). *The Three Worlds of Welfare Capitalism*. Princeton, NJ: Princeton University Press.

Esping-Andersen, G. (1999). *Social Foundations of Postindustrial Economies*. Oxford: Oxford University Press.

Ghilarducci, T. (2007). *Guaranteed Retirement Accounts: Toward Retirement Income Security*. Economic Policy Institute, Agenda for Shared Prosperity. Washington, D.C.

Gran, B.K. (2003). A second opinion. *International Journal of Health Services, 33*(2), 283–313.

Hacker, J. (2002). *The Divided Welfare State*. Cambridge: Cambridge University Press.

Hinrichs, K. and Kangas, O. (2003). When is a change big enough to be a system shift? *Social Policy and Administration*, 37(6), 573–591.

Keeley, B. (2014). *The Measure of Poverty. OECD Insights*. Accessed December 31, 2015: http://oecdinsights.org/2014/06/30/the-measure-of-poverty.

OECD (2013). *Pensions at a Glance 2013: Retirement-income Systems in OECD and G20 Countries*. Paris: OECD.

OECD (2015a). *Global Pension Statistics*. Paris: OECD.

OECD (2015b). *Pensions at a Glance: Retirement-income Systems in OECD and G20 Countries*. Paris: OECD.

OECD (2015c). *OECD Statistics—Income Distribution and Poverty: By Country—Inequality*. Paris: OECD.

OECD (2015d). *Income Distribution and Poverty: By Country—Poverty (Poverty Line: 50%)*. Paris: OECD.

OECD Working Party on Private Pensions (2005). *Private Pensions: OECD Classification and Glossary*. Paris: OECD.

Overbye, E. (1997). Mainstream pattern, deviant cases: The New Zealand and Danish pension systems in an international context. *Journal of European Social Policy*, 7(2), 101–117.

Pierson, P. (2001). *The New Politics of the Welfare State*. New York: Oxford University Press.

President's Commission to Strengthen Social Security (2001, December 21). *Strengthening Social Security and Creating Personal Wealth for all Americans: The Final Report of the President's Commission to Strengthen Social Security*. Accessed: http://govinfo.library.unt.edu/csss/reports/Final_report.pdf.

Rohter, L. (2006, January 10). Chile's candidates agree to agree on pension woes. *New York Times*, January 10. Accessed: www.nytimes.com/2006/01/10/international/americas/10chile.html?ex=1294549200&_r=0.

Rowlingson, K. (2002). Private pension planning: The rhetoric of responsibility, the reality of insecurity. *Journal of Social Policy*, *31*(4), 623–642.

Schwartz, H. (2001). Round up the usual suspects! In P. Pierson (ed.), *The New Politics of the Welfare State* (pp. 17–44). New York: Oxford University Press.

St. John, S. and Gran, B. (2001). The world's social laboratory: Women friendly aspects of New Zealand pensions. In J. Ginn, D. Street and S. Arber (eds), *Women, Work and Pensions*. Buckingham: Open University Press.

Turner, J.A. and Rajnes, D. (2014). Social security and pension trends around the world. In M. Szczepański and J.A. Turner (eds), *Social Security and Pension Reform: International Perspectives* (pp. 13–36). Kalamazoo, MI: W.E. Upjohn Institute for Employment Research.

United Nations Development Programme (2015). *Income GINI Coefficient*. Accessed December 31, 2015: http://hdr.undp.org/en/content/income-gini-coefficient.

World Bank (1994). *Averting the Old Age Crisis*. Washington, DC: Oxford University Press for the World Bank.

World Bank (2015). *GINI Index*. Accessed December 31, 2015: http://data.worldbank.org/indicator/SI.POV.GINI.

12 Grey ghettos

Inclusion or exclusion in the post-modern Canadian city?

Gina Sylvestre and Nora Cristall

The promotion of opportunities for seniors to age in place and remain vital and active in their community involves material, individual, community and environmental factors. To advance understanding within this scope, we consider the experience of growing old in an urban milieu that we identify as a *grey ghetto*, that is: an impoverished community occupied by older adults predominantly living in material and social disadvantage. With a conceptualization of spheres theorized to impact inclusion and exclusion of seniors in the inner city mosaic, our study utilized participatory action research methods to engage key informants in drawing their knowledge and obtaining feedback regarding the introductory framework. Our subsequent enhanced framework is introduced in this chapter with the ultimate goal to more systematically recognize the threats to social inclusion for the older population in the post-modern Canadian city.

There is growing interest in supporting seniors in their community with numerous strategies to assist the older adult in remaining independent and in their own community for as long as possible. Many seniors become isolated while at the same time wanting to stay in a familiar neighborhood, attending established organizations and maintaining everyday activities. In our study of a grey ghetto, we examine the challenges to maintain independence and the engagement of seniors across the spheres of material resources, the neighborhood, services and programs, the community and the individual. In this discussion, we pay particular attention to the risks of exclusion for seniors living in poverty and discuss the specific effects of income benefits and the social safety net impacting Canadian seniors. We place this discussion in the context of the inner city of Winnipeg, Manitoba, by first introducing you to the historical urban context and then to the post-modern city. So much can be learned about the inner city of a metropolis, by first going back to the heritage of the urban centre, in this case Winnipeg's North End community.

Winnipeg's North End: islands of inclusion

A deep social and economic division has existed since the early history of Winnipeg, spatially segregating the poor and ethnically marginalized populations of the city (Silver, 2006; Werner, 2007). The infamous North End of Winnipeg was originally a multicultural enclave of Jewish, Ukrainian, German and Polish immigrants who were able to create an "island of inclusion" by sustaining their cultural heritage in the midst of an exclusionary dominant British elite. More recently, the ghettoizing processes of the postmodern city hastened the neglect of Winnipeg's inner city, perpetuating the exclusion of both older immigrants and newly arrived Canadian Indigenous groups. The once unified North End has been fragmented into isolated islands of inclusion.

The development of the Canadian Pacific Railway mainline reflected the early economic boom of Winnipeg, but the railway line and station became a physical barrier between the North End and the city's central and southern areas. "North of the Tracks" came to represent the boundary between the privileged and powerful British and those less tolerated based on differing cultural practices and religious beliefs (Gourluck, 2010). The Higgins underpass built in 1904 was one of the few suitable crossings that connected two distinct realities (Figure 12.1). Immigrants from Eastern Europe came to fill the many jobs available with the advancement of the railroad and industrialization, but their meagre pay relegated them to the separate world of newcomers (Werner, 2007).

Originally the North End was coined the "New Jerusalem," but, as the Jewish population moved further north and south of the tracks, they were replaced by consecutive waves of Ukrainians, Germans and Poles, thus framing the area as the foreign section of the city (Gourluck, 2010). The arrival of large numbers of immigrants resulted in rapid construction of poorly built housing on small lots rarely connected to sewer and water lines, and with few provisions for parks and recreational spaces. The low wages of the occupants of these homes lead to overcrowding, unsanitary conditions, undernourishment and frequent moves. Unacceptable living conditions have been the continued reality of the North End until today (Silver, 2006).

Despite impoverished living conditions, the North End became distinguished as an epicentre of cultural inclusion amongst a populace with similar lifestyles, beliefs and traditions. Synagogues, churches and voluntary associations were organized to preserve religious and social traditions, while mutual aid societies supported individual members in times of illness, death and unemployment (Grenke, 1991). There were newspapers in several European languages, music and drama societies, as well as literary associations and sports clubs. The Ukrainian Labour Temple, built on McGregor Street in 1912, housed a print shop and a 1,000-seat theatre supporting political activities, drama and music groups, along with language and folkloric dance instruction (Gourluck, 2010; Yuzyk, 1953). The heart of the North End was a flourishing commercial district on Selkirk Avenue where the various immigrant groups found familiarity in the ethnic diversity of the goods offered and the languages spoken. Kosher butcher shops intermingled with German delis, women's fashion and hardware stores. The

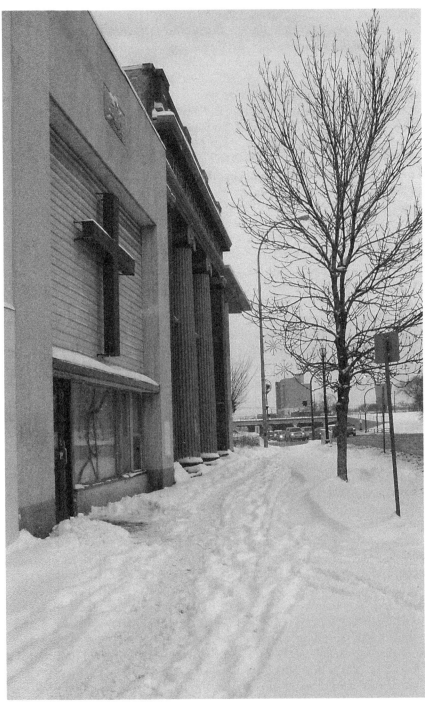

Figure 12.1 Main Street at Higgins looking north to the CPR mainline tracks

Saturday morning market was considered a social mecca within the North End (Gourluck, 2010). The cultural and commercial vibrancy of the North End created pride and a strong sense of community in this multicultural realm (Silver, 2006).

This refuge of inclusion began to change dramatically after World War II when the processes of suburbanization prompted the descendants of original immigrants to leave the North End for new homes and larger lots. The houses left behind were taken over by slum landlords whose quest for profit allowed the housing stock to deteriorate (Gourluck, 2010). The demise of the once-thriving commercial life of Selkirk Avenue soon followed as businesses either shut down or moved to growing suburban locations (Silver, 2006). Ultimately, the rich social and cultural life of the North End deteriorated as churches and cultural associations began to close.

The North End became the destination for new waves of international immigrants from the Caribbean, the Philippines and India seeking low-cost housing similar to the experience of those who had arrived earlier (Werner, 2007). It was also in this period that Indigenous Canadians began to migrate to metropolitan centres and they soon became the largest growing ethnic group in Winnipeg's inner city (Kives, 2014). These new urban dwellers became the next targets of discrimination, leaving them vulnerable to slum landlords and social exclusion (Silver, 2006). In the North End of today, there is a ghettoizing of the poor, excluded from mainstream housing and forced into overcrowded conditions in sub-standard housing that precipitates constant residential transiency (Distasio et al., 2013).

Currently, these city-level exclusionary processes continue, but the North End has become a landscape of exclusion itself, divided by disparate islands of inclusion particularly for the aging population. Poverty and inequality have always been deeply entrenched in the North End and this post-modern inner city is now renowned for crime, violence and gang activity with a backdrop of derelict and abandoned housing along with pawnshops and payday loan establishments (Gourluck, 2010) (Figure 12.2). Where previously neighbors knew one another and no one locked their doors, now elderly residents are afraid to leave their homes (Silver, 2006).

In the midst of these isolating processes, however, there are signs of economic and cultural renewal that are less formal and based on grass roots, community-driven initiatives. Non-profit organizations and informal neighborhood volunteers have replaced the original mutual aid agencies. Improvements are also supported by the presence of European delicatessens and bakeries, as well as Indigenous food cooperatives and credit unions. Educational and social service agencies now occupy many of the storefronts on Selkirk Avenue (Gourluck, 2010). While these may represent distinct islands of inclusion, concern for the older population is notably absent as most initiatives are focused on youth and families. Nonetheless, the continuing existence of the Ukrainian Labour Temple and the German Society are signs of the North End's original immigrant cultures (Figure 12.3). Our

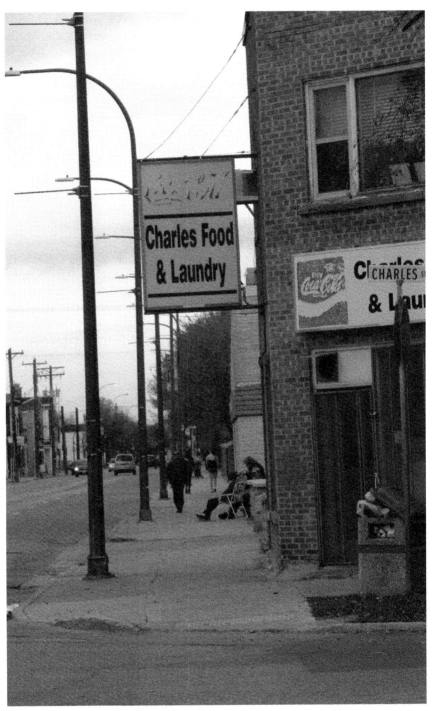

Figure 12.2 Streetscape of Selkirk Avenue

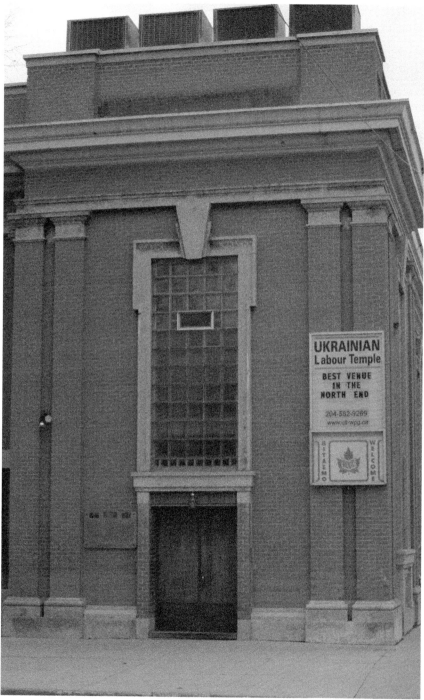

Figure 12.3 Ukranian Labour Temple

study seeks to understand how these distinct islands of inclusion impact aging in Winnipeg's North End.

Habitus: framing aging in Winnipeg's North End

We began this investigation with a curiosity to understand the paradox between the North End's rich cultural heritage and conflicting current realities by walking in the neighborhoods, talking to seniors about their memories and experience with growing older during the advent of the post-modern ghetto. We also secured input from care providers in both the informal and formal sectors to inform our process. Through this immersion, we refined a conceptual framework to examine the extent of inclusion–exclusion in what we found to be the grey ghetto of Winnipeg's inner city. Our framework draws from the sociological theory of Bourdieu's *habitus* (Bordieu, 1984) and his explanation of the importance of heritage and historical memories of groups as part of the evolution of people's behavior and social interaction. We also introduce the concepts of *cultural structuralism* and *social capital* presented by Bourdieu (1984, 1993) as they help contextualize the involvement of elders in the post-modern urban city centre.

French Philosopher Pierre Bourdieu introduced a theoretical foundation that we refer to and build on as he provides an important backdrop to understand groups of people and how the individual and the group are influenced by each other. In his description of the habitus, Bourdieu offers critical underpinnings to ask why there are embedded practices and beliefs and an acceptance of class, gender and other socially contrived power differences in people's everyday lives (Bourdieu, 1984). As he explains, there is often an entrenched acceptance of the dominant narrative in how societies are organized and what is valued and who is, and who is not, part of the social group.

Dominant structures such as government services and formal education are recognized as static. Assuming objective markers such as social class and gender role expectations are fixed and unchanging in the process of cultural structuralism, Bourdieu describes the way formal organizations and systems reinforce this dominant paradigm (Bourdieu, 1984). This organizing field determines how people within the formal structure participate and are eligible for civic engagement, with the habitus informing behavior and roles within the social setting. This behavior is often predetermined and reinforced by the organizing principles that influence expectations and relationships that are reproduced within the community and wider social structure (Bourdieu, 1993).

Bourdieu also provides an important concept in understanding people's motivations and behaviors in what he describes as social capital. That is, acquiring and disbursing non-material resources that can be expended when needed to maintain ones well-being and status in the area. This is important at all ages but social contact and support become vitally important as people grow older. Through the life course, people acquire material advantage and they also acquire social capital. That is, social contacts and influence that they can expend when they need to.

Bourdieu's habitus represents the conceptual basis for our consideration of social and economic inclusion as it sets the narrative of power differences, valuing and devaluing specific groups within the organization of society. Building on this foundation, we developed and tested a typology to evaluate inclusive processes. With findings from our investigation, we present our framework for examining the inclusion–exclusion continuum proposing five spheres that are dynamic in nature with both interactive and dimensional forces supporting islands of inclusion. This framework provides a starting point to operationalize Bourdieu's theory and examine the extent of inclusion at the neighborhood, community, program and services, material and individual levels (Figure 12.4).

The framework focuses first on the sphere of material resources as the adequacy of income and food security are primary determinants to attain satisfactory participation within the larger context of the post-modern city.

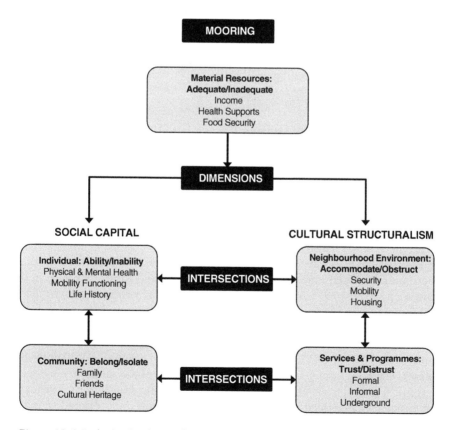

Figure 12.4 Inclusion/exclusion framework of aging

As Levitus (2005) emphasizes, if these resources are far below average, the individual is excluded from what are considered to be normal activities and customs of society. We view material resources to be the mooring for the remaining four spheres.

The structure of the inclusion–exclusion framework proposes two relational dimensions. First, the spheres of the individual and the community encompass the social resources that are paramount to the existence of social capital. The health, functioning and life history of aging individuals influence their ability or inability to engage, while the role of family, friends and cultural heritage determine their experience of isolation or belonging. Second, aspects that reinforce the power paradigm of cultural structuralism are encompassed in our framework's spheres of neighborhood environment and services and programs. The neighborhood accommodates or obstructs seniors' inclusion depending upon the quality of housing, mobility and safety. Furthermore, the range of formal, informal and underground supports in the neighborhood promote trust or distrust of the aging population, ultimately affecting inclusionary processes of the social network.

Using the knowledge gained from key informant interviews, our understanding of the proposed intersections and dimensional qualities of the framework was extended. The following section outlines, first, the methodology of the study and, second, how our key findings contributed to a more comprehensive understanding of the dynamics of the spheres in creating both inclusion and exclusion in a grey ghetto.

The inclusion–exclusion continuum: the experience of aging in a grey ghetto

With participatory action qualitative methodology, we found the inclusion–exclusion framework to be a tenable way of contextualizing how elderly communities structure opportunities for engagement and connections. This inquiry allowed for the active participation of key informants, interacting both formally and informally to participate in the framework development. Their knowledge and expertise was imperative as they "have a rich knowledge of the local neighbourhood that can be used to safeguard the continuation of planning across the past, present, and future" (Verma and Huttunen, 2015, p. 97). The participatory inquiry gave them an active voice and ongoing participation in the study design, direction and interpretation of findings (Dominelli, 2016; Reason, 1994).

The evolution of our framework involved in-person interviews in the summer and fall of 2015 with 18 key informants representing a variety of roles in the community, including housing, health and community service settings. A primary element of participatory action research is the cyclical dimensions that enabled our participants to reflect on the proposed framework, provide commentary and additional context and ultimately confirm the conceptual structure that is presented here (Kindon et al., 2007).

This inquiry guided us in the evolution of the framework with five spheres that illustrate the experiences of inclusion and exclusion for older adults. The purpose of this discourse is to demonstrate that while exclusionary processes are part of a grey ghetto, distinct islands of inclusion mediate the effects of neglect for an aging population. In the next section, we highlight key observations and give examples of processes across the framework spheres.

Material resources

Material resources influence inclusion and exclusion across the tensions of privilege and disempowerment. When advancing into senior years, material resources and access to adequate goods and services enhance inclusion or contribute to social exclusion and isolation. Unfortunately, there has been little or no attention to economic considerations in age-friendly frameworks or initiatives to date (Menec et al., 2012; Steels, 2015). Income sources and the extent of a social safety net separates older adults from other age groups and also marginalizes populations of older adults who receive subsistence-level benefits. The key informants emphasized that experiencing low income throughout life is problematic in old age, particularly for those who did not contribute to a private pension plan or the Canada Pension Plan (CPP). This most often applies to people who received income assistance benefits or were newly arrived immigrants. Older adults who have become widowed and single seniors are especially vulnerable to having minimal disposable income in old age (Bazel and Mintz, 2014). These are formal structures that influence many aspects of daily living and limit active participation for sectors such as the aging population.

Older adults subsisting on small pensions represent a dehumanizing process overlooked by most Canadians. There are limited options for housing with subsidized senior housing concentrated in undesirable areas such as Winnipeg's North End. Those seniors who lack funds but remain in their own homes often live in sub-standard conditions with broken windows and lack of insulation. Low-income seniors have little opportunity for leisure activities or any other quality-of-life enhancing past times. These in turn become isolating factors and impact disparity in power and privilege.

It is difficult to pursue a healthy lifestyle when living in poverty. Despite universal access to healthcare in Canada, there are many resources that are not covered. This includes third party benefit plans such as Pharmacare in Manitoba, a provincial drug program that covers the expense of medication on a sliding income-based scale. Some individuals are unable to pay the deductible, compromising their spending choices when considering medication expenses. Key informants revealed that many aging individuals ration or share their prescription medications. Other medical needs without coverage include prescriptions glasses, dentures, walkers and even ambulance services. It was suggested that a lack of access to these resources creates a reliance on an underground system of bartering.

Food security is also a concern as many key informants spoke of older adults who ran out of food before their next pension cheque was due. An important revelation of this study was that Winnipeg Harvest, the largest food bank supplier in Winnipeg, does not allow food to be delivered to those with mobility limitations. This suggests that many seniors living in poverty go without sufficient food, particularly in the winter months when sidewalks can be icy and impassable.

Overall, our findings confirm that the sphere of material resources is the determining factor of exclusion as the lack of adequate funds for housing, healthcare and food access impacts all facets of life for older persons. In the following sub-sections, the intersections of the remaining framework spheres illustrate that material resources influence all other spheres, limiting social capital and, in other ways, promoting the cultural structuralism of power.

The individual and the neighborhood environment

Individual attributes influence inclusion as some individuals are more outgoing and have the capacity to maintain social networks and contacts, while others are more naturally prone to being alone or not participating. In older age, these personal characteristics can be barriers to successful integration, especially if someone needs to make changes in their social network (Vanderbeck, 2007). Loneliness is a major challenge that increases with age and isolation is associated with decreasing health, depression and an increased mortality risk (Verma and Huttunen, 2015). Loneliness can be a personal issue related to depression or decreased self-care that is reinforced by fewer monetary resources, an inaccessible built environment and an unsafe surrounding area.

Individual attributes influence the extent of social inclusion by empowering the individual to engage in adequate self-care and remain independent. The framework proposes that one's ability to maintain self-care is related to health status and functional mobility. The key informants spoke repeatedly of the issue of cognitive decline and its impact on self-neglect. For example, a neighbor, concerned about an older man's decline following the onset of dementia, contacted a service provider who was unable to assist because the individual refused help. This man was still living in his own home, unaware of his circumstances despite broken windows in the middle of winter and his inability to access food.

Many participants explained how declining health, disability, low self-esteem, addictions and anger issues promote isolation. A community facilitator discussed the challenge of isolation and the self-exclusion of older adults who are prevented from interaction because of cognitive decline. He also spoke about the isolation from care of Indigenous seniors in particular who may be aware of their mental health issues, but self-exclude because life experiences have created distrust of the formal helping system.

Apart from age-related barriers to individual empowerment, a senior's life history may also affect exclusionary processes. Despite the island of inclusion created by the entrenched cultural practices of European ethnic groups, historically, there is an inherent distrust of government leadership emanating from their experiences of anti-Semitism, Russian oppression and lack of religious freedom (Gourluck, 2010; Yuzyk, 1953). The Indigenous peoples that replaced the first generations of Eastern European immigrants are similarly marginalized. Their mistrust of mainstream society stems from the long history of colonialism, racism, segregation on reserves and the residential school system leading to a loss of cultural identity (Distasio et al., 2013).

It was also postulated by a participant that cultural-related barriers affect one's interaction with the neighborhood environment. The life history of a person is associated with their familiarity and sense of security in the community. If memories are positive about the place where their life was built, an older person will find comfort in continued immersion in that milieu, and, as one informant noted, will adapt better to changes related to the aging process. The early multicultural history of the North End provides a reference point for aging European immigrants who continue to seek identity within their cultural group. Conversely, if memories relate to exclusionary processes, the senior may be less inclined to remain an active member of that neighborhood.

Individual attributes of health and functioning also impact an older person's ability to interact in the community. This environment influences the extent of inclusive processes by providing age-friendly and accessible community attributes that either accommodate or obstruct participation (Burns et al., 2011; Scharf et al., 2005). Accessible places that provide thriving public access and green space will have more flourishing residents who are able to walk freely in safe areas (Verma and Huttunen, 2015). The same is true for a more impoverished physical environment, in which case the environment can limit how much people want to go out, how far they will go and opportunities for active participation. A tenant resource coordinator spoke about the importance of green space but that tenants of the seniors' block were reluctant to walk to parks because of perceived danger. Similarly, they knew other areas of the neighborhood to avoid and did not go out at night.

The physical environment also impacts inclusion considering the location of local community stores, coffee shops and other places where people connect. If older persons are unable to walk or have access to a car, they are less likely to get acquainted with a community of people that may offer peer support and cultural activities (Scharlach and Lehning, 2013). This can inhibit the development of the habitus and acquisition of social capital. In the North End, seniors are limited from full participation because of insufficient spaces for community gatherings, uneven sidewalks that are icy in the winter and the lack of benches for resting.

A further important resource for older persons is the availability of healthy foods in grocery stores. The North End has an abundance of expensive corner stores, but full-service grocers fled the deteriorating community long ago. One example of a grass-roots initiative that has created an island of inclusion is a free weekly grocery bus that is run by an anonymous philanthropist and coordinated by the North End Renewal Corporation. The shuttle brings multiple generations and ethnic groups to big-box stores for access to more economical food prices. It represents neighborhood trust and networking, with some seniors participating mainly for the social outing.

Access to affordable and appropriate housing is another important asset. Key informants noted that housing in the inner city is often in ill repair and unsuited to older residents. There are forgotten seniors, for example, living on the third floor of a house and having to share a bathroom on the second floor. Subsidized senior housing offers aging individuals with physical and social supports that promote community; however, such housing in the area is in ethnic-based complexes. Our informants indicate that strong religious and cultural ties in existing communities such as the Ukrainian and Polish groups contribute to social inclusion with established senior-enriched housing close to churches and other cultural outlets. St. Mary the Protectress, for example, is attached to a Ukrainian Orthodox church that continues to be the centre for social, spiritual and cultural activities (Figure 12.5). The Polish Manor on Selkirk Avenue is across the street from a Polish Catholic church, while this housing complex includes a Polish restaurant and grocery store, as well as Polish library books and television. Seniors from these established cultural communities are more likely to provide mutual support and ensure the well-being of all housing tenants, uniting many residents who spent their youth and adulthood in Winnipeg's North End.

The community and services and programing

Along with individual attributes, characteristics of the community also inform the extent of inclusion. In the community, there are those more informal sources of social support that sustain vibrancy in an area. There is a large component of community involving cultural activities and integration of the past and continued participation in normative activities (Phillipson, 2007). Cultural identification throughout the lifespan creates communities of support for individuals.

Community cultural heritage contributes to the habitus by informing the roles and behaviors of groups. This influences social capital; how social influence is expended. Social capital can be as important as monetary resources in maintaining the independence of the elderly for as long as possible. Part of both inclusion and social capital is being part of and supported by a community of people. Community assistance includes the extent of integration families provide to the elder to assist with advocacy when necessary and access to goods and services as well as social interaction (Gardner,

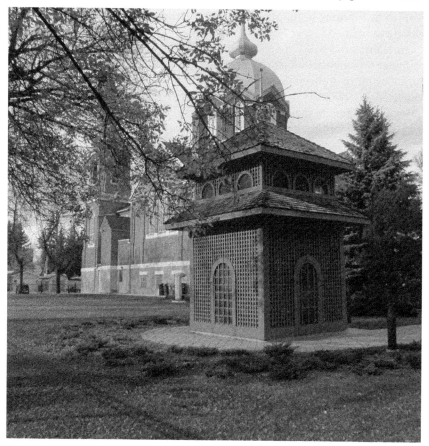

Figure 12.5 St. Mary the Protectress Ukrainian Orthodox Church and Millennium Villa

2011; Vanderbeck, 2007). Informants indicated that when family support exists, seniors do not require extensive formal supports.

The European-based population has experienced an exodus of educated adult children to the suburbs and out-of-province, creating a cavity of close regular contact for older adults. On a tour of the area, a life-time resident pointed out several homes of childhood friends where declining parents remained isolated from community integration with a lack of formal supports. Seniors recall when everyone spoke to one another, but the present neighborhood mix of the North End often includes families that are not familiar to the senior residents, reinforcing distrust and safety concerns.

In contrast, informants spoke about the more active lifestyle of Indigenous seniors included in a community of extended families. These seniors contribute to child-care and promote traditional knowledge, such as bannock making. However, the legacy of colonialism has also created family dysfunction and the addiction issues of younger generations can unfortunately lead to disruptions in the senior housing setting and financial abuse of the elderly individual.

In many large western Canadian cities, there is recognized systemic discrimination against Indigenous people. Participants recognized this barrier to inclusion of Indigenous seniors as there are vast differences in cultural expectations regarding extended family, with Indigenous residents often having other family members stay overnight in the senior's complex. There was an explanation that specific Indigenous elders were well integrated in community activities and liked, as individuals, but as a group there is mutual distrust that separates residents within the community.

Isolation from the community also occurs for those Indigenous individuals who have been transient between the home community and city, or who have moved to Winnipeg in old age because of medical needs. For these seniors, KeKiNan Senior Housing offers an island of inclusion where tenants look out for one another and the tenant resource coordinator attempts to provide cultural connections for this marginalized group. However, the lack of cultural- and language-inclusive services for these seniors acknowledges widespread cultural structuralism practices within formal and informal organizations and institutions.

The composition of services and programs impacts how and in what ways seniors participate in the civic, social and cultural activities in the area. In this sphere, there are challenges in providing the most suitable services for seniors and targeting those who can benefit most. Many poverty-reduction strategies and intervention programs often target lone parents and children in programing, with the rationalization that breaking the cycle of poverty happens at the family level.

There was agreement by many of the key informants that services and programs offered to the older population in the North End are inadequate because of a range of factors, including language barriers, little integration with the dominant group, minority status and systemic discrimination. In some instances, inequality is perpetuated, as service provision is inadequate when compared to other parts of Winnipeg. Homecare, for example, is limited for those who live in unsafe areas, rooming houses or do not have family members who can provide a backup resource (Martens et al., 2007). In the case of Age and Opportunity's friendly visitor program for socially isolated seniors, the North End is excluded entirely because of lack of volunteers.

Key informants expressed frustration at the systematic barriers they face in the North End to address the social isolation experienced by older adults. On many occasions, the inadequacy of the healthcare system was emphasized specifically surrounding gaps in services for mental health. One tenant resource coordinator spoke of going to the hospital to facilitate with clinicians care for one of her tenants who did not have family and was found wandering by the train tracks. Other examples were also found of service providers committed to overcoming barriers by advocating for seniors and seeking appropriate services.

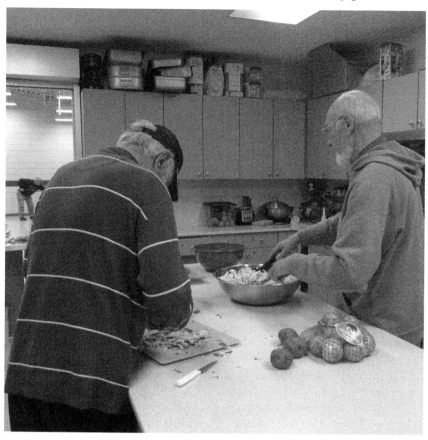

Figure 12.6 Volunteers at the North End Seniors Wellness Program preparing lunch

Overall, the exploration of formal services and programs in the North End confirmed that cultural structuralism exists, creating distinct experiences for those aging in poverty. One island of inclusion was found, however, at the informal level. The North End Seniors Wellness Program is run entirely by volunteers to create a "second home" for older adults to meet for socialization and midday meals (Figure 12.6). This informal group also provides rides to members to participate in programs at a recreational centre and ensures that they have transportation to medical appointments. To address the exclusionary processes that exist in a grey ghetto, it is imperative for the formal sector to begin to partner with such informal services. However, there is still a great deal to be learned about networks of support in a grey ghetto as the tenant resource coordinator at KeKiNan Senior Housing has discovered that underground circuits exist to obtain needed resources, but as an outsider, it is difficult to access this community.

Conclusion: creating inclusion

Despite the growing needs of older adults living in poor neighborhoods, exploration of the nature of poverty and exclusion for seniors continues to be underexplored (Scharf et al., 2005). The social and ecological restructuring occurring in post-modern metropolises is creating new realities of inclusion and exclusion for inner-city populations, yet the consequences of socio-spatial marginalization have not been considered from the perspective of aging (Phillipson, 2004; Sylvestre, 2015). Age-friendly development requires consideration at multiple spatial levels (Verma and Huttunen, 2015). As well, creating more inclusive environments requires cross-sector collaboration with specific attention to the unique attributes of the cultural groups and heritage within the area. Bringing forward history and tradition provides continued opportunities for social networking, civic engagement and belonging in inner cities that are balancing modernization with tradition.

Our key informants provided important observations and recommendations to support inclusive environments for seniors. A primary innovation is adequate income replacement and equitable access to services. Although Canada has been an international leader in pension benefits, approximately 5 percent of senior Canadians are below the low-income cut-off, yet for single elderly women who live alone, close to 20 percent have income replacements that were below the low-income cut-off in 2012 (Bazel and Mintz, 2014). Current federal pension benefits continue to leave a group of Canadians with an income that is substantially lower than the low-income cut-off for the area (Bazel and Mintz, 2014). Pension and income assistance programs do not provide enough benefits to help all Canadians to afford basic necessities. Also, safe neighborhood environments require adequate mobility resources, public spaces and opportunities for community meals. In addition, programing must target the most marginalized, specifically addressing mental health issues that create isolation and exclusion.

Building on Bourdieu's theory, we were able to provide an expansive framework that identifies key components of inclusion. We found that many disparate islands of inclusion exist, with limited integration for a large number of inner-city seniors. The "waters" are not stable and exclusion in reality represents complex processes with barriers across spheres that inhibit inclusion. Innovation and multi-sector initiatives are necessary to make aging in place a reality. Further research involving key sectors should ideally guide innovation.

This research can direct continued participatory enquiry with input to affect change in policy in a variety of urban settings. We plan to continue the refinement of the framework with ongoing input from key informants and seniors living in the area. In this kind of enquiry, it is important to examine opportunities for input from harder-to-reach populations, such as seniors living at home and those who are transient and precariously housed. It would be valuable to test this framework in other inner-city communities and in the context of other urban areas with a large proportion of senior residents. It is vital to continue to capture the stories and lived experiences of seniors grappling with social integration and tenure in a familiar environment. We found this to be a valuable collaborative research environment across geography and social work that expanded the view of both disciplines. Innovative collaborations are necessary to inform policy and practice for our aging populations.

References

Bazel, P. and Mintz, J. (2014). Income adequacy among seniors: Helping singles most. *School of Public Policy SPP Research Papers*, 7(4), 1–17.

Bourdieu, P. (1984). *Distinction*. London: Routledge.

Bourdieu, P. (1993). *The Field of Cultural Production: Essays on Art and Literature*. New York: Columbia University Press.

Burns, V.F., Lavoie, J.P. and Rose, D. (2011). Revisiting the role of neighbourhood change in social exclusion and inclusion of older people. *Journal of Aging Research, 2012*, 1–13.

Distasio, J., Sylvestre, G. and Wall-Whieler, E. (2013). The migration of First Nations peoples in the Canadian Prairie context: Exploring policy and program implications to support residential stability. *Geography Research Forum, 33*, 38–63.

Dominelli, L. (2016). Participatory action research: Empowering women to evaluate services. In L. Hardwicke, R. Smith and A. Worsley (eds), *Innovations in Social Work Research: Using Methods Creatively*, 274–294. London: Jessica Kingsley.

Gardner, P.J. (2011). Natural neighbourhood networks: Important social networks in the lives of older adults aging in place. *Journal of Aging Studies, 25*, 263–271.

Gourluck, R. (2010). *The Mosaic Village*. Winnipeg, MB: Great Plains Publications.

Grenke, A. (1991). *The German Community in Winnipeg, 1872–1919*. New York: AMS Press.

Kindon, S., Pain, R. and Kesby, M. (2007). Introduction: Connecting people, participation and place. In S. Kindon, R. Pain and M. Kesby (eds), *Participatory Action Research Approaches and Methods: Connecting People, Participation and Place*, 1–6. New York: Routledge.

Kives, B. (2014). The "great indigenous divided": Winnipeg stares into an ethnic chasm. *The Guardian*, October 21.

Levitus, R. (2005). *The inclusive Society? Social Exclusion and New Labour*, 2nd edn. Basingstoke: Palgrave Macmillan.

Martens, P.J., Fransoo, R., Burland, E., Burchill, C., Prior, H.J. and Ekuma, O. (2007). Prevalence of mental illness and its impact on the use of home care and nursing homes: A population-based study of older adults in Manitoba. *Canadian Journal of Psychiatry*, 52(9), 581.

Menec, V.H., Hutton, L., Newall, N., Nowicki, S., Spina, J. and Veselyuk, D. (2015). How "age-friendly" are rural communities and what community characteristics are related to age-friendliness? The case of rural Manitoba, Canada. *Ageing & Society, 35*(1), 203–223.

Phillipson, C. (2004). Urbanisation and ageing: Towards a new environmental gerontology. *Ageing & Society, 24*, 963–972.

Phillipson, C. (2007). The "elected" and the "excluded": Sociological perspectives on the experience of place and community in old age. *Ageing & Society*, 27, 321–342.

Reason, P. (1994). Three approaches to participatory inquiry. In N. Denzin and Y. Lincoln (eds), *Handbook of Qualitative Research*, 324–339. Thousand Oaks, CA: SAGE.

Scharf, T., Phillipson, C. and Smith, A.E. (2005). Social exclusion of older people in deprived urban communities of England. *European Journal of Ageing*, 2, 76–87.

Scharlach, A.E. and Lehning, A.J., (2013). Ageing-friendly communities and social inclusion in the United States of America. *Ageing & Society*, 33(1), 110–136.

Silver, J. (2006). *North End Winnipeg's Lord Selkirk Park Housing Development: History, Comparative Context, Prospects.* Winnipeg, MB: Canadian Centre for Policy Alternatives.

Steels, S. (2015). Key characteristics of age-friendly cities and communities: A review. *Cities*, 47: 45–52.

Sylvestre, G. (2015). Ageing in Winnipeg's inner city: Exclusion or inclusion in polarized urban spaces? In J. Distasio and A. Kaufman (eds), *The Divided Prairie City: Income Inequality Among Winnipeg's Neighbourhoods, 1970–2010*, 62–67. Winnipeg, MB: Institute of Urban Studies, University of Winnipeg.

Vanderbeck, R.M. (2007). Intergenerational geographies: Age relations, segregation and re-engagements. *Geography Compass*, 1/2, 200–221.

Verma, I. and Huttunen, H. (2015). Elderly-friendly neighbourhoods: Case lauttasaari. *Journal of Housing for the Elderly*, 29(1–2), 92–110.

Werner, H. (2007). *Imagined Homes: Soviet German Immigrants in Two Cities.* Winnipeg, MB: University of Manitoba Press.

Yuzyk, P. (1953). *The Ukrainians in Manitoba: A Social History.* Toronto, ON: University of Toronto Press.

13 What drives older consumers' entertainment choices?

Gord Hendren, Gillian Joseph and Kristin Crawford

In recent years, Canadians have increased their Internet usage, with over 90 percent of them currently accessing or subscribing to Broadband at home (Colledge and Tong, 2015). However, researchers continue to remind us that we cannot generalize when it comes to adopting digital technology, because different groups of people have different patterns of use (Veenhof and Timusk, 2007). In a survey undertaken in 2010, 60 percent of Canadians aged 65–74 indicated that they had used the Internet. However, in that same year, only 10 percent of those 65 or over reported that they watched movies or videos on the Internet compared to almost 80 percent of their counterparts aged 18–24 years (Allen, 2013).

Baby Boomers (Boomers), defined in Canada as people born between 1945 and 1964, represent the "younger" older adults whose patterns of technology use may be quite different to those of older cohorts (Wagner et al., 2010). For example, in the United States, only 24 percent of Boomers own smartphones, but they represent the fastest growing segment of smartphone owners (Sabi, 2015). Furthermore, nearly 35 percent of tablet owners in the United States are over the age of 45 (Sabi, 2015). Yet the media often portrays Boomers and other older adults as lacking in technological capabilities despite the fact that many Boomers used CP/M, DOS or even Unix operating systems long before Macs and PCs had graphical user interfaces—and some older adults even built their own computers from scratch (Magid, cited in Stein, 2013). As the number of older adults who are comfortable using digital technology increases, its use for the purpose of leisure and entertainment has grown rapidly (Lee, 2012). Keeping in mind the importance of not generalizing across groups, our focus in this chapter is on exploring how Canadian Boomers use technology for entertainment purposes. Specifically, we examine their use of digital video content through TV and mobile devices.

Over the past 70 years, Boomers have lived through unprecedented levels of change within the entertainment industry (Brown, 2015). From nickel theatres to multiplexes, black-and-white televisions to 4K Ultra HD monitors, three channels to hundreds, the options for Boomers to engage with video content has grown rapidly. Yet, despite the fact that Boomers were the first cohort of children to be studied as consumers (Sabi, 2015), their patterns of technology use and opinions on viewing preferences are not always sought by hardware manufacturers or software developers (Brown, 2015). Rather, marketing companies often focus on the purchases and practices of younger, seemingly more tech-savvy, consumers (Lee and Coughlin, 2014). This may make some sense from a marketing perspective because it has been shown that younger people not only purchase technology for themselves but also influence the technological spending habits of their parents and teachers (Poulton, 2008; Wadhwa, 2014). Yet as the number of older consumers continues to increase worldwide, the lack of information about their digital viewing preferences creates a widening gap in our understanding of the economic impact of this rapidly growing sector of the entertainment market (Lee and Coughlin, 2014).

Beyond the economic implications, the gap in knowledge about the older technology consumer is also an important concern in a social and political sense (Russell and Young, 2015). For example, as governments, financial organizations and other sectors increasingly move away from paper-based documentation in favor of more digitally-based, paperless communication, understanding the "how" and "why" associated with access and use of digital technology will become crucial. Answering these questions will not only identify critical barriers associated with adoption, but it may also uncover solutions to problems and dispel myths associated with negative attitudes that marginalize older adults and prevent them from engaging fully in democratic, social and economic processes that shape the quality of everyday life (Russell and Young, 2015).

Researchers also point out that technology is not a benign tool, but one that interacts with its user in ways that can facilitate physiological changes, invite certain social behaviors and even define the spaces in which consumers are required to act (Aceros et al., 2015). For example, in the physiological sense, it has been shown that older adults who use certain digital technologies repetitively, experience mental stimulation in parts of the brain that improves decision making, complex reasoning and memory (Small et al., 2009; Xavier et al., 2014). In a social sense, the use of technology helps older adults to live independently longer and to maintain control over important aspects of their own lives as they age. Older adults gain greater social capital by connecting with family and friends on Facebook, Skype or e-mail, and can obtain information about staying healthy or how to manage their resources more effectively (Russell and Young, 2015). Moreover, engaging with online technology provides a sense of accomplishment that positively correlates with well-being. For example, Cotten et al. (2014) found that Internet use contributed to the mental well-being of retired adults, especially those living alone. As well-being improves, demand for and costs of government resources go down. Thus, information about the use of technology may help to reveal the extent and intricacies of these reciprocal processes.

Finding ways to narrow the gaps in information about older adults and technology use will not only make technology more relevant, useful and marketable to older consumers, but it may also assist in dispelling myths that incorrectly generalize about the abilities of older adults (Aceros et al., 2015). There are many examples of older adults who are firmly linked to technological innovation. For example, Canadian Graeme Ferguson and his team members were over the age of 40 when they invented the IMAX theatre system. Stephanie Kwolek was 41 when she invented Kevlar, a very strong material that is used today in cell phones and drones. Even Steve Jobs, widely known as the CEO of Apple computers, who contributed to the development of the iMac, iTunes, iPod, iPhone and iPad, did so after the age of 45 (Wadhwa, 2011). When older adults are characterized as less physically and mentally competent, change aversive and less adaptable, these attitudes become internalized so that even older adults themselves begin to believe that they cannot learn new things (Magsamen-Conrad et al., 2015). For older adults who want to engage with technology, derogatory attitudes that ignore their needs and preferences sets old against young in an ageist spiral. Therefore, to ignore how older people use technology is to create what Peine et al. (2015) call "triple jeopardy": older people will not get what they need, markets will not realize the full potential of an aging consumer and government subsidies will misalign—creating policies and prototypes that waste resources.

We continue with a brief review of the history of entertainment technology and then outline the Theory of Planned Behavior that is used as a theoretical touchstone in the analysis. The Research Process section outlines data collection methods and describes the characteristics of the sample. The Results and Discussion sections are followed by the Conclusion that brings together the main points and speculates on how Boomers will use entertainment technology in the future.

Looking back

Ever since our distant ancestors entertained themselves by poking a stick into a termite hill, technology has been an important part of life for people of all ages. In fact, some would argue that since humans are the weakest of all primates—with vulnerable eyes, fragile backs and infantile helplessness—it was technology and not natural selection that compensated for our deficiencies and pushed us down an evolutionary path distinct from other animals (Taylor, 2010).

As practical as technology has been through the ages, it has also provided us with stimulating opportunities for leisure. Ng (2012) describes the complex path of innovation that led to digital entertainment technologies. Thomas Edison created the first entertainment machine, the phonograph, in 1877. This device was able to record voice or music onto a disk which could then be moved to another location and played back to a larger group of people. The pioneers of the radio industry also understood the benefits of entertaining larger groups at one time (Ng, 2012). Louis Lumière, followed by Thomas Edison, was instrumental in the development of moving pictures. After the first television was demonstrated in 1927, technology associated with communicating sight and sound to even larger audiences developed rapidly. By the 1960s, as Boomers were growing up, cable became the preferred means of TV distribution, providing a number of channels and programs.

In the 1970s, the demand for higher quality in both sound and picture pushed the entertainment industry forward. CDs and DVDs were the first digital entertainment products, and satellite TV followed shortly after. When the United States moved from analog television broadcasting to digital in 2009, portable technology in the form of mobile devices was quick to come to market. Today, video media is the most popular source of digital entertainment (Ng, 2012).

By definition, video media includes half-hour TV comedies, hour-long TV dramas, short films, educational videos, documentaries, independent films and summer blockbusters—anything that can be accessed with a movie, television, computer, tablet or smartphone screen. There is now a plethora of video content viewing options for the purpose of entertainment and a number of theories have been developed to assist in explaining user adoption preferences.

A theoretical lens

Although the Theory of Planned Behavior is not tested formally in this study, its basic concepts are useful as a "touchstone" to assist in the interpretation of findings. Originally developed by Icek Ajzen in 1985, the theory suggests that technology use is determined by three factors: (1) *attitudes toward IT use*, which suggests that the more positively the technology is perceived, the more likely it will be used; (2) *subjective norms about its use*, which includes whether people who are important to the user think he or she should engage in the behavior; and (3) *perceived control over use*, or self-efficacy, that includes the extent that the user feels she/he is able to use the technology, or believes that the goal of using the technology will be realized (Ajzen, 1985; Knabe, 2012).

The Theory of Planned Behavior has been used to understand the adoption of technological innovations in numerous quantitative and qualitative studies. For example, Morris and Venkatesh (2000) used the theory to study workers' attitudes and decisions about technology adoption. The theory has been used as a way to better understand the use of technology in the professional arenas of social work and nursing (Kondo and Ishida, 2014; Zhang and Gutierrez, 2007) and online teaching (Lee et al., 2010). More recently, the theory has been used in studies that explore online entertainment (Kondo and Ishida, 2014; Troung, 2009; Lee and Tsai, 2010). We expand upon this growing body of literature on technology adoption by connecting the concepts of the Theory of Planned Behavior to a new focus on Baby Boomers and their use of digital video entertainment technologies (Knabe, 2012). To our knowledge, this link has not been made before.

The research process

The data for this study come from research conducted in 2014 by Charlton Strategic Research, Inc. located in Toronto, Ontario, Canada, on behalf of the Cable and Telecommunications Association for Marketing (CTAM) Canada. It focuses specifically on Digital Video Consumption.

The goal of our study was to answer the following research questions: (1) how have Canadian Baby Boomers adapted to changes in accessing digital video content and (2) how does their behavior differ from the generations that followed them? With all of the different options available, the study also sought to understand (3) what are the means through which Boomers are choosing to access video content?

Using standard market research practice, an online survey was conducted in June 2014 of 3,062 Canadians aged 18 or older. The sample was sourced from a national panel and weighted to be representative of Canadian households in terms of age, gender and region.

The aggregate Boomer subsample consists of a total of 1,188 adults who were aged 50–69 at the time of the survey. This was broken down further into two subgroups, the first aged 50–59 (n=566) and the second aged 60–69 (n=622). The younger adult group consists of a total of 1,874 adults aged 18–49. This younger cohort is also broken down further into two subgroups, one aged 35–49 (n=1,017), which approximates a demographic group called *Generation X* that follows the Boomer generation, and a second aged 18–34 (n=857), which approximates a demographic group called *Millennials* who were born in the last two decades of the twentieth century.

Findings

This section reports the main findings of the research in three parts. *General video content consumption* reports on the time that Boomers spend watching video content, their user preferences, the reasons they choose not to use other viewing options available to them and the video genre that is most important to them. *Perceptions of Paid TV service* highlights the main findings about the content viewing option most preferred by Boomers, and *Over-the-top & TV everywhere* describes Boomers' perspectives of online services. All differences cited below are statistically significant.

General video content consumption

There are two main ways that video content can be accessed. The first is through Paid TV subscription (for example, using digital cable, analog cable, satellite TV or internet protocol TV) and the second is by what is called "over-the-top" content (OTT) which refers to content that arrives from a third party—such as Hulu, Netflix, Sling TV or WhereverTV (Gonçalves et al., 2010).

As shown in Figure 13.1, in 2014 Boomers spent a great deal of time, on average 32.9 hours per week, watching video content. This was significantly more than among 18–49 year olds, who watched only 25.5 hours per week on average.

> Question: Of all the programing you watch, indicate how many hours you spend watching in the following ways during a typical week.

Boomers indicate that they spend most of their viewing time watching video content on a television screen using a paid subscription. In fact, Boomers are more likely than 18–49 year olds to have a Paid TV subscription, particularly digital or analog cable. That being the case, it is not surprising that Boomers spend more money per month on television subscriptions than do 18–49 year olds on average ($68.90 per month versus $57.43 respectively). However, it is interesting to note that Boomers spend the highest proportion of their video content viewing with a Paid TV subscription during the show's scheduled time (18.8 hours per week on average), with the second highest proportion watching pre-recorded video content with a Paid TV subscription using a digital video recorder (DVR) (6.3 hours per week on average). In contrast, Boomers spend only 6.9 hours per week, or only 21 percent of their total viewing time, watching video content away from

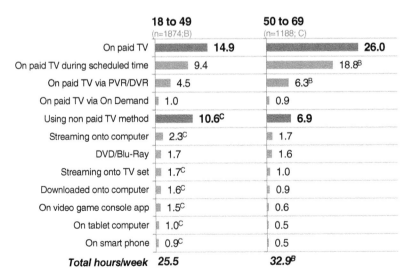

Figure 13.1 Hours spent watching video content per week

a Paid TV subscription. This is much lower than among 18–49 year olds, who spend 10.6 hours per week on average watching away from a Paid TV subscription, or 42 percent of their total viewing time.

Among Boomers, the most frequently stated reasons for not watching content online was that "it is too complicated" or they "do not know where to look." In contrast, for 18–49 year olds who do not watch content online, "low resolution in online video content" or a "lack of time to watch content at all" are the most frequent reasons for not watching content online.

It is interesting to note that *what* Boomers watch is very different to the content viewed by their younger counterparts, and this can be seen in something as basic as Boomers' preferred video content genres. When asked what TV genres they consider "must haves" for their household, Boomers are much more likely to answer "news and information" or "nature and science" and are less likely than 18–49 year olds to identify "music," "family," "children/pre-school," or "comedy" as "must-have" genres. Thinking specifically about the importance of the "news and information" genre, Generation X and Millennials differ from Baby Boomers in that they prefer so-called "entertainment journalism" programs such as *The Daily Show with Trevor Noah*, *The Colbert Report* or *Last Week Tonight with John Oliver* for their news. They are also far more likely than Boomers to go online for news content, where dozens—if not hundreds—of news sites, blogs and social media personalities provide up-to-the-minute coverage of the biggest stories of the day.

Perceptions of Paid TV service

As previously mentioned, Canadian Boomers are more likely than 18–49 year olds to have a Paid TV subscription. In fact, 94 percent of Boomers subscribe to some form of Paid TV, whether it be digital cable, analog cable, satellite TV or some other form of paid service.

Question: Have you changed TV service providers in the past year?

Question: Have you ever considered reducing your TV subscription package?

Question: Have you ever considered cancelling your TV subscription package and not having any kind of TV subscription?

Among those who do subscribe, as noted in Figure 13.2, Boomers also demonstrate a higher degree of loyalty to their subscription provider than 18–49 year olds. Despite the amount of upheaval in the communication industry in recent years, Boomers are more likely to say they are very satisfied with their TV provider, less likely to have changed TV providers in the past year and less likely to consider trimming the number of channels they subscribe to or cancelling their subscription entirely. It is also interesting to note that

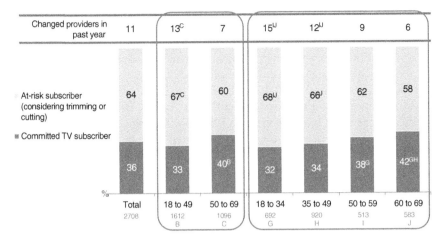

Figure 13.2 TV subscription loyalty among current subscribers

Boomers who currently subscribe are much more likely than 18–49-year-old subscribers to strongly agree that they "do not know how they would get by without a Paid TV subscription." Along those same lines, Boomers are also less likely to agree they "see little need for a TV subscription" or they "do not need a TV subscription, as they can find everything they want online."

> Question: Please indicate how strongly you agree or disagree with the following statements about cable/satellite service subscription.

However, as noted in Figure 13.3, Boomers' perceptions of Paid TV are not entirely positive. The growing number of channels available today is actually viewed negatively by Boomers, who are much more likely than 18–49 year olds to *strongly* agree that "TV packages include too many channels they're not interested in."

Over-the-top and TV everywhere

As happened earlier with the music industry, video content has become increasingly available online via OTT services. As noted above, OTT services include both licensed, for-pay methods (e.g. Netflix) and unlicensed, for-free sites (e.g. Pirate Bay). As may be expected, given that they spend less time watching video content away from Paid TV, Boomers are less likely than 18–49 year olds to own or subscribe to, or even be aware of, any of the OTT services tested in 2014 as noted in Figure 13.4.

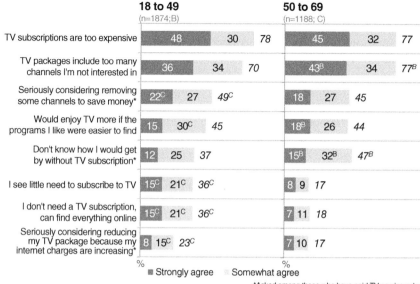

Figure 13.3 Perceptions of Paid TV service

| | 18 to 49(B) | | | 50 to 69(C) | |
	Aware	Own/Subscribe		Aware	Own/Subscribe
Any (NET)	93^C	57^C		91	36
Netflix	89^C	43^C		85	22
Smart TV	72^C	19^C		67	14
Apple TV	67^C	11^C		48	7
Xbox Live	64^C	13^C		45	3
Google Play	50^C	8^C		36	3
Playstation Network	44^C	12^C		37	2
Roku	25^C	4^C		16	2
Chromecast	26^C	4^C		17	1
Amazon Instant Video	22^C	3^C		15	0

Figure 13.4 Awareness of and subscription to OTT services

Question: Have you heard of the following devices/services before this survey?

Question: Which of the following devices, if any, do you currently own/ subscribe to?

Looking specifically at Netflix, a subscription-based service that has offered video content via home-delivered DVDs or online streaming since 1997 and has millions of subscribers worldwide, only 22 percent of Boomers said they subscribed to it in 2014. In contrast, among 18–49 year olds, 43 percent said they subscribed to Netflix. However, interestingly, among those who do subscribe to Netflix, Boomers report similar levels of satisfaction and likelihood to continue their subscription as do 18–49 year olds.

Surprisingly, Boomers are just as likely as younger cohorts to be aware of TV apps and websites offering video content. As shown in Figure 13.5, they are also just as likely to be aware of the TV Everywhere (TVE, ways to watch paid TV content on devices other than TV) options being provided by television service providers. One could speculate that Boomers are knowledgeable about all of the TVE products because they are more likely to be TV subscribers who watch commercials and are therefore more likely to be exposed to advertising about these services. Despite this awareness, when asked about actually *using* these services, Boomers hesitate. They are less likely to use the TV apps and websites listed on the survey and indicate a lower degree of interest in the TVE options tested. Only 21 percent of Boomers rate their interest in using TVE as "eight to ten out of ten" in comparison to 28 percent of 18–49 year olds who chose the same rating. Furthermore, 30 percent of Boomers rate their interest in using TVE as "one

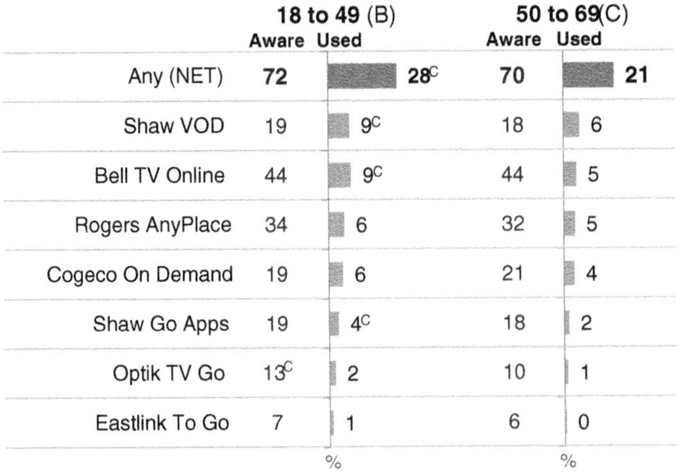

	18 to 49 (B)		50 to 69 (C)	
	Aware	Used	Aware	Used
Any (NET)	72	28^C	70	21
Shaw VOD	19	9^C	18	6
Bell TV Online	44	9^C	44	5
Rogers AnyPlace	34	6	32	5
Cogeco On Demand	19	6	21	4
Shaw Go Apps	19	4^C	18	2
Optik TV Go	13^C	2	10	1
Eastlink To Go	7	1	6	0
	%		%	

Figure 13.5 Awareness and use of TVE services

to three out of ten," compared to only 21 percent of 18–49 year olds who chose the same rating.

> Question: Have you heard of the following services before this survey?

> Question: Which, if any, of the following services have you used before?

Discussion

As noted earlier, one way to conceptualize Boomers' comfort with and use of video content consumption is by connecting the findings to the concepts of the Theory of Planned Behavior. By linking the theoretical framework to our results, it may be possible to better understand how and why Boomers adopt, or do not adopt, the video content viewing options that are available to them. However, it is important to keep in mind that the concepts of this theory are more complicated than our analysis might suggest. Nevertheless, linking our findings to the theoretical concepts of the theory, even at this basic level, provides insights that highlight where stronger influences may lie.

Beginning with hours spent watching video, we see that Boomers not only spend more time watching video content than do younger groups, but they also predominantly watch TV through a paid subscription. However, Boomers are also more likely to indicate that they feel that Paid TV packages include too many channels that hold little interest for them. If Boomers' critical attitudes about Paid TV influence their proclivity for watching it, then the theory would suggest that their disapproval of too many channels should result in either choosing options other than Paid TV or increasing their use of DVR recorders to view only the content that they find interesting. Yet our findings suggest that Boomers watch more scheduled-time Paid TV content than any other viewing option, despite this criticism. Moreover, watching pre-recorded video content via DVR only represents 6.3 hours of viewing per week on average for this group. Therefore, contrary to the theory, Boomers' negative attitudes to the overwhelming number of channels available does not appear to influence their preference for viewing content via Paid TV.

How Boomers are influenced by others in their preferences, integral to the *subjective norms* aspect of the theory, does not seem to be straightforward. Our data show that Boomers are less likely than their younger counterparts to want to have the newest technology before their friends, or to be the first to learn about a new website. However, because Boomers in general are less likely to use online services and newer technologies than other groups, it might be speculated that older adults who do not use certain technologies are influenced by this fact. On the other hand, contrary to the theory, the fact that Boomers are less likely to compete with their peers to have the latest technology might also suggest a cohort effect—that competing with peers to have the latest technology is not as important to Boomers as it is to their younger counterparts.

When we look at reasons why Boomers do not watch content online, we see a stronger connection to the theory. Boomers most frequently state that they find watching content online as "too complicated" or they "do not know where to look." This fits with the *perceived control* concept of the theory that suggests that people will not adopt technology if they believe that they will not be able to master it. It may also explain why a majority of Boomers are not interested in the more complicated TVE viewing options, even though they are aware of them. However, although Boomers are less likely than younger groups to view content via OTT services such as Netflix, Boomers who *do* subscribe to OTT services report similar levels of satisfaction and the same likelihood to continue services as do their younger counterparts. This suggests that should Boomers become more comfortable using technologies either through training or by developers improving the user-friendly qualities of the products, Boomers' perception of control will be enhanced and they will be more likely to adopt the technology, perhaps even to the same extent as younger groups. When it comes to Boomers' preferences for content viewing then, our results suggest that for some Boomers, *perceived control* may outweigh *attitude* and *subjective norms* in influencing and predicting video content viewing choices.

One of the reasons why younger people might be more knowledgeable of, and comfortable using, new technologies may be the fact that they are learning about and using them regularly in schools at the same time as they are using them at home (Magsamen-Conrad et al., 2015). Having constant access to technology and the knowledge of how to use it enhances user confidence. Researchers have found that although seniors expressed anxiety about using new technologies and computers, it was their tendency to underestimate their ability and knowledge about how to use them that contributed most to their stress (Mitzner et al., 2010). This supports our findings on the influence of *perceived control* and the potentially dominant role it may play in shaping technology adoption by Boomers. Mitzner et al. (2010) suggest that teaching older adults how to use technology would provide them with more confidence and, in particular, give clear information about how specific technologies can benefit older adults' needs to be part of that educational strategy.

As suggested earlier, ageism is a factor that has been shown to affect learning about technology (Peine et al., 2015). When people are constantly bombarded with media images and articles about the technological incompetence of older adults, younger and older people internalize these stereotypes and make erroneous assumptions that can affect the desire to learn and adopt.

Conclusion and looking ahead

Since prehistoric times, technology has been an important part of human life. Research has shown that for older adults in particular, learning about and using new technologies contributes to a sense of well-being, helps to maintain independence and keeps people connected to their communities, both socially and politically. Filling the gap in knowledge about technology preferences and use can help us to better understand how technology shapes physiological, social and behavioral systems. Research has shown that using technology can be very beneficial for older adults, specifically in terms of age-related cognitive change and building social capital. Studies suggest that older adults enjoy using new technology—if they find it useful, if people in their networks encourage them and if they gain confidence to tackle the learning curve. In this regard, the Theory of Planned Behavior is a useful tool for gaining a better understanding of how and why older adults engage, or do not engage, with digital entertainment technology.

Predominantly, Boomers access video content through Paid TV subscription and at the program's scheduled time. Furthermore, despite dissatisfaction with the service and contrary to what is proposed by the theory, Boomers maintain their loyalty to Paid TV, pay more for it than their younger counterparts and even believe that they could not get by without it.

Reasons why Boomers do not want to watch content online include their perception that it is too complicated to access, or their belief that they do not know where to look for it. This finding is in line with the Theory of Planned Behavior's concept of perceived control, suggesting that confidence and self-efficacy may be strong predictors of technology use for Boomers.

As they were growing up, Boomers watched assassinations, wars, royal weddings, Olympics and humanity's first steps on the moon on their television screen. It's no wonder, then, that they continue to view content on television and prefer "news and information" and "nature and science" content as their key genres. Since Boomers spend more time watching video content using a Paid TV service, and considering they saw the birth of in-home subscriptions, it follows that Boomers have a very different relationship with Paid TV than do younger Canadians.

As to how methods of video content consumption will continue to change, the music industry is an instructive model that helps us to speculate on the future. The rise of "grey market" websites (legal, but used for purposes beyond what was intended by the developer), such as the controversial Pirate Bay, can be seen as a parallel to the outdated Napster service for the music industry such that younger Canadians were quick to take advantage of free online options to access their preferred content. After unsuccessful attempts by content-makers, service providers, regulatory boards and even governments to shut down these sites, it can be observed that newer, officially-licensed sites have stepped in to fill the same desire for content, without infringing on copyright or breaking other laws.

In what is perhaps the clearest reflection of the parallel story between the music and video content industries, we see that several online services such as iTunes and Amazon are serving both industries. As the music industry eventually discovered, many young Canadians are willing to pay for content as long as it is easily available when and where they want it, they don't have to pay for content they don't want and it is at a reasonable price. For Boomers, this trend toward affordable and flexible online content means that increasingly there is greater pressure to shift to online viewership. There are already television series available only online, with sites such as Netflix, Amazon and Hulu now producing their own content. Although most of that content has been targeted toward younger age groups, it may only be a matter of time before high-profile, award-winning content is only available through OTT services.

When reflecting upon Boomers' dissatisfaction with overwhelming channel options, pick and pay subscriptions may be of interest to some who would like to streamline their packages. However, pick and pay subscription models can be more complicated, which may deter some people.

Another digital entertainment genre, this one unique to the video content industry, is that of live sport events. Unlike most television programing that can be enjoyed at any time after its initial airing, sporting events are still considered "appointment viewing," best enjoyed as they happen. For television providers, this means that sport networks such as TSN, Sportsnet and ESPN have been heavily promoted as reasons to subscribe to Paid TV. However, this too may soon change. TSN and Sportsnet both offer TV Everywhere-style websites and apps so that Paid TV subscribers can watch this content online. At the same time, sport leagues such as Major League Baseball and the National Hockey League offer content direct to their fans through online-based subscription services, avoiding the need for a TV subscription. Although the vast majority of live games are still exclusive to Paid TV channels, online options may continue to grow.

Fortunately, Boomers are well-practiced at adapting to change, as their life experience suggests. Furthermore, it won't be long until younger cohorts face their own challenges associated with adopting ever-changing technological innovation as they age. As history has shown, the number of different ways that Boomers can engage with video content is growing, and, as they become more comfortable with these options, their adoption rates may increase. As long as there is video content worth watching and a screen on which to view it, it is more than likely that Canadian Boomers will be there.

References

Aceros, J.C., Pols, J.D. and Domenech, M. (2015). Where is grandma? Home telecare, good aging and the domestication of later life. *Technological Forecasting & Social Change*, 93, 102–111.

Ajzen, I. (1985). From intentions to actions: A theory of planned behavior. In J. Kuhl and J. Beckmann (eds), *Action Control: From Cognition to Behavior*. Berlin, Heidelberg/New York: Springer-Verlag, pp. 11–39.

Allen, M.K. (2013). *Consumption of Culture by Older Canadians on the Internet.* Ottawa: Statistics Canada.

Brown, R.L. (2015, January 15). *Canada's Baby Boom is Nothing Like the One in the U.S.* Huffington Post blog. Retrieved from www.huffingtonpost.ca/robert-l-brown/canada-baby-boom_b_6478760.html.

Colledge, M. and Tong, G. (2015). *One in Ten (9%) Canadians Do Not Have Internet Access at Home.* Toronto: Ipsos Reid.

Cotten, S.R., Ford, G., Ford, S. and Hale, T.M. (2012). Internet use and depression among older adults. *Computers in Human Behavior, 28*(2), 496–499.

Gonçalves, V., Evens, T., Alves, A.P. and Ballon, P. (2014). *Power and Control Strategies in Online Video Services.* Paper presented at the 25th European Regional Conference of the International Telecommunications Society (ITS), Brussels.

Knabe, A. (2012). *Applying Ajzen's Theory of Planned Behavior to a Study of Online Course Adoption in Pubic Relations Education.* Doctoral disertation. Marquette University, Milwaukee, Wisconsin. Retrieved from http://epublications.marquette.edu/cgi/viewcontent.cgi?article=1186&context=dissertations_mu.

Kondo, F. and Ishida, H. (2014). A cross-national analysis of intention to use multiple mobile entertainment services. *Journal of Global Information Technology Management, 17*, 45–60.

Lee, B. (2012). Cyber behaviors among seniors. In Z. Yan (ed.), *Encyclopedia of Research on Cyber Behavior.* Hershey, PA: IGI Global, pp. 233–239.

Lee, C. and Coughlin, J.F. (2014). Older adults' adoption of technology: An integrated approach to identifying determinants and barriers. *Journal of Product Innovation Management, 32*(5), 747–759.

Lee, J., Cerreto, F.A. and Lee, J. (2010). Theory of planned behavior and teachers' decisions regarding use of educational technology. *Educational Technology & Society, 13*(1), 152–164.

Lee, M.C. and Tsai, T.R. (2010). What drives people to continue to play online games? An extension of technology model and theory of planned behavior. *International Journal of Human-Computer Interaction, 26*(6), 601–620.

Magsamen-Conrad, K., Dowd, J., Abuljadail, M., Alsulaiman, S. and Shareefi, A. (2015). Life-span differences in the uses and gratifications of tablets: Implications for older adults. *Computers in Human Behavior, 52*, 96–106.

Mitzner, T.L., Boron, J.B., Bailey Fausset, C., Adams, A.E., Charness, N., Czaja, S.J., Dijkstra, K., Fisk, A.D., Rogers, W.A. and Sharit, J. (2010). Older adults talk technology: Technology usage and attitudes. *Computers in Human Behavior, 26*, 1710–1721.

Morris, M. and Venkatesh, V. (2000). Age differences in technology adoption decisions: Implications for a changing work force. *Personnel Psychology, 53*, 375–403.

Ng, S. (2012). A brief history of entertainment technologies. *Proceedings of the IEEE: 100. Special Centennial Issue,* pp. 1386–1390.

Peine, A., Faulkner, A., Yaeger, B. and Moors, E. (2015). Science, technology and the "grand challenge" of ageing: Understanding the socio-material constitution of later life. *Technological Forecasting and Social Change, 93*(April), 1–9.

Poulton, T. (2008, February 22). Kidfulence' on family spending strong: YTV Report. *Media in Canada.* Retrieved from http://mediaincanada.com/2008/02/22/tweenreport-20080222.

Russell, H. and Young, K. (2015). Influences and experiences of using digital devices in laterlife. *Journal of Community Informatics*, *11*(1). Retrieved from http://ci-journal.net/index.php/ciej/article/view/1008/1129.

Sabi (2015). *The Boomer Report*. Sabi. Retrieved from www.slideshare.net/jah2183/boomers-4-may15smallbook.

Small, G.W., Moody, T.D., Siddarth, P. and Bookheimer, S. (2009). Your brain on Google: Patterns of cerebral activitation during internet searching. *American Journal of Geriatric Psychiatry*, *17*(2), 116–126.

Stein, J. (2013, January 29). It's stupid and insulting to pitch baby boomers as tech novices. *Forbes*. Retrieved from www.forbes.com/sites/jonstein/2013/01/29/2013-the-year-your-grandpa-becomes-more-tech-savvy-than-you/#1141f27f78bf.

Taylor, T. (2010). *The Artificial Ape: How Technology Changed the Course of Human Evolution*. London: St. Martin's Press.

Troung, Y. (2009). An evaluation of the theory of planned behaviour in consumer acceptance of online video and television services. *Electronic Journal of Information Systems Evaluation*. *12*(2), 197–206.

Veenhof, B. and Timusk, P. (2007). *Online Activities of Canadian Boomers and Seniors*. Ottawa: Statistics Canada.

Wadhwa, V. (2011, December 2). The case for old entrepreneurs. *Washington Post*. Retrieved from www.washingtonpost.com/national/on-innovations/the-case-for-old-entrepreneurs/2011/12/02/gIQAulJ3KO_story.html.

Wadhwa, V. (2014, November 9). Why baby boomers will rule the future of technology. *Daily Herald*. Retrieved from www.highbeam.com/doc/1G1-389537573.html.

Wagner, N., Hassanein, K. and Head, M. (2010). Computer use by older adults: A multi-disciplinary review. *Computers in Human Behavior*, *26*, 870–882.

Xavier, A.J., d'Orsi, E., de Oliveira, C.M., Orrell, M., Demakakos, P., Biddulph, J.P. and Marmot, M.G. (2014). English longitudinal study of aging: Can internet/e-mail use reduce cognitive decline? *Science Medical Sciences*, *69*(9), 1117–1121. Retrieved from http://biomedgerontology.oxfordjournals.org/content/69/9/1117.full.

Zhang, W. and Gutierrez, O. (2007). Information technology acceptance in the social services sector context: An exploration. *Social Work*, *52*(3), 221–231.

Index

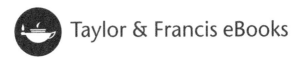

Printed and bound by CPI Group (UK) Ltd, Croydon, CR0 4YY

24/10/2024

01778306-0003